Dental Public Health
at a Glance

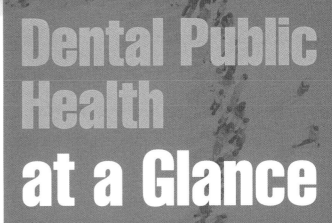

Dental Public Health
at a Glance

Ivor G. Chestnutt

BDS, MPH, PhD, FDS (DPH) RCSEdin, DDPH,
FDS RCSEng, FDS RCPSGlas, FFPH, FHEA
Professor and Honorary Consultant in
Dental Public Health
School of Dentistry
Cardiff University
Cardiff
UK

WILEY Blackwell

This edition first published 2016 © 2016 by John Wiley & Sons, Ltd

Registered office: John Wiley & Sons, Ltd, The Atrium, Southern Gate, Chichester, West Sussex, PO19 8SQ, UK

Editorial offices: 9600 Garsington Road, Oxford, OX4 2DQ, UK

The Atrium, Southern Gate, Chichester, West Sussex, PO19 8SQ, UK

1606 Golden Aspen Drive, Suites 103 and 104, Ames, Iowa 50010, USA

For details of our global editorial offices, for customer services and for information about how to apply for permission to reuse the copyright material in this book please see our website at www.wiley.com/wiley-blackwell

The right of the author to be identified as the author of this work has been asserted in accordance with the UK Copyright, Designs and Patents Act 1988.

Designations used by companies to distinguish their products are often claimed as trademarks. All brand names and product names used in this book are trade names, service marks, trademarks or registered trademarks of their respective owners. The publisher is not associated with any product or vendor mentioned in this book. It is sold on the understanding that the publisher is not engaged in rendering professional services. If professional advice or other expert assistance is required, the services of a competent professional should be sought.

The contents of this work are intended to further general scientific research, understanding, and discussion only and are not intended and should not be relied upon as recommending or promoting a specific method, diagnosis, or treatment by health science practitioners for any particular patient. The publisher and the author make no representations or warranties with respect to the accuracy or completeness of the contents of this work and specifically disclaim all warranties, including without limitation any implied warranties of fitness for a particular purpose. In view of ongoing research, equipment modifications, changes in governmental regulations, and the constant flow of information relating to the use of medicines, equipment, and devices, the reader is urged to review and evaluate the information provided in the package insert or instructions for each medicine, equipment, or device for, among other things, any changes in the instructions or indication of usage and for added warnings and precautions. Readers should consult with a specialist where appropriate. The fact that an organization or Website is referred to in this work as a citation and/or a potential source of further information does not mean that the author or the publisher endorses the information the organization or Website may provide or recommendations it may make. Further, readers should be aware that Internet Websites listed in this work may have changed or disappeared between when this work was written and when it is read. No warranty may be created or extended by any promotional statements for this work. Neither the publisher nor the author shall be liable for any damages arising herefrom.

Library of Congress Cataloging-in-Publication Data

Names: Chestnutt, I. G., author.

Title: Dental public health at a glance / Ivor G. Chestnutt.

Other titles: At a glance series (Oxford, England)

Description: Chichester, West Sussex, UK ; Ames, Iowa : John Wiley & Sons, Inc., 2016. | Series: At a glance | Includes bibliographical references and index.

Identifiers: LCCN 2015043947 (print) | LCCN 2015044762 (ebook) | ISBN 9781118629406 (paper) | ISBN 9781118629376 (pdf) | ISBN 9781118629390 (epub)

Subjects: | MESH: Public Health Dentistry—Handbooks. | Dental Health Services—Handbooks. | Oral Health—Handbooks.

Classification: LCC RK56 (print) | LCC RK56 (ebook) | NLM WU 49 | DDC 617.6—dc23

LC record available at http://lccn.loc.gov/2015043947

A catalogue record for this book is available from the British Library.

Wiley also publishes its books in a variety of electronic formats. Some content that appears in print may not be available in electronic books.

Cover image: © Tai11 / Shutterstock

Set in 9.5/11.5pt Minion Pro by Aptara Inc., New Delhi, India

Printed and bound in Singapore by Markono Print Media Pte Ltd

1   2016

Contents

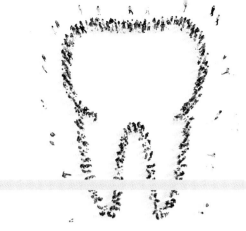

Preface

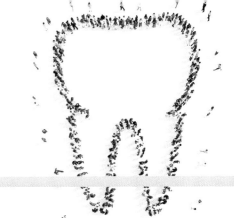

Members of the dental team are in a unique position to offer tailored and personalized advice and to thereby educate their patients on the steps that are necessary to secure oral health. However, there is only so much that can be achieved by such one-to-one, 'downstream' interventions. It is crucial that all members of the dental team appreciate the wider determinants of health and the impact of lifestyle and life circumstances on the health and oral health of their patients. The population has not benefited equally from the significant improvements in oral health observed over the past four decades. That one half of all diseased teeth are concentrated in just 7% of 5-year-olds serves to highlight the health inequalities that pervade our society. It is crucial that from the earliest stage of their training, the next generation of dental professionals have an appreciation that the lives of others are frequently very different from their own.

Dental students rightly spend the majority of their time learning the theoretical, practical and clinical skills necessary to practise their chosen profession. Often it is only relatively late in their course that their attention turns to the environment in which they will have to deliver dental care and earn their living. It is important to have an appreciation of the issues involved in the organization, commissioning and delivery of oral healthcare at dental practice, regional, national and international levels. The principles of evidence-based practice are of ever-increasing significance in achieving this. In its guidance *Preparing for Practice*, the General Dental Council has placed great emphasis on learning outcomes that fall within the remit of dental public health. All of these factors emphasize the need for an understanding of the discipline.

The intention of this book is that 'at a glance' dental professionals will be able to come to a basic understanding of the principles and practice that relate to the science and the art of improving oral health at both an individual and a population level. Of course, the factors influencing public health practice evolve at a pace – a change of government, new guidance and new policies affect dental public health at a greater rate than other dental specialties. For this reason, the intention of this book is to raise awareness and provide pointers and flags that can be followed up via more exhaustive information sources.

While the basic principles of the discipline are universal, a complicating factor in writing a book on dental public health in the United Kingdom is the four different – sometimes very different – models of care that have evolved in the constituent countries following devolution in 1999. Where possible, attempts have been made to illustrate differences across the United Kingdom, but at times this is limited by the constraints of space.

The primary audience for this book is undergraduate dental, dental therapy and dental hygiene students, together with those in Dental Foundation and Core training and those preparing for MDFS or MJDF examinations. The book should also prove a useful resource for those preparing for the Diploma in Dental Public Health examination or the Overseas Registration examination. While at an entry level, the book may also act as an aide mémoire for those undertaking specialty training, and may indeed be of use to any member of the dental team who has an interest in the vast range of topics now embraced within dental public health.

The concepts arising in dental public health can be challenging from an academic perspective. Twenty years teaching the subject have taught me that it is one that students tend to love or hate. It is my hope that this book might go some way to encouraging more of the former and less of the latter.

I.G. Chestnutt
Cardiff
April 2015

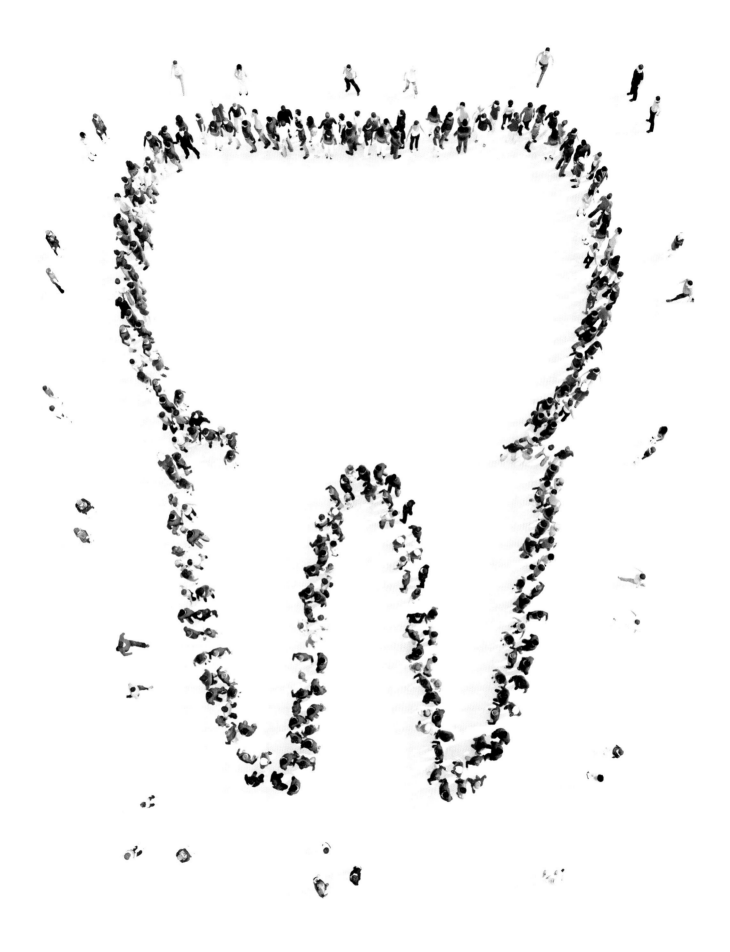

Introduction

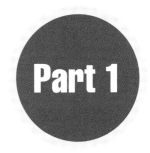

Part 1

Chapters

What is dental public health?

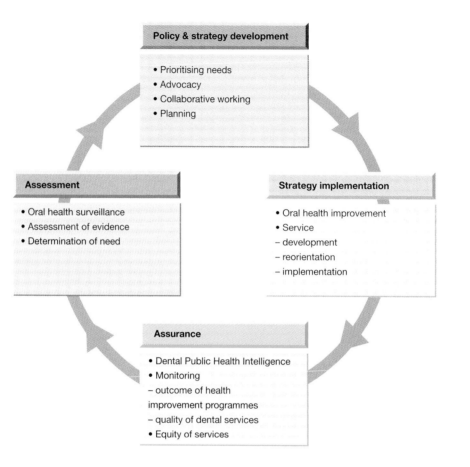

Figure 1.1 Components of Dental Public Health Practice

Policy & strategy development
- Prioritising needs
- Advocacy
- Collaborative working
- Planning

Assessment
- Oral health surveillance
- Assessment of evidence
- Determination of need

Strategy implementation
- Oral health improvement
- Service
  - development
  - reorientation
  - implementation

Assurance
- Dental Public Health Intelligence
- Monitoring
  - outcome of health improvement programmes
  - quality of dental services
- Equity of services

*D*ental public health is the science and the art of preventing oral disease, promoting oral health and improving the quality of life through the organized efforts of society.

In contrast to clinical dental practice, where the focus is on looking after individual patients, in dental public health practice the focus is on populations or defined groups within a population. The definition here refers to **science**. Dental public health requires a sound knowledge of the factors influencing the aetiology, detection, measurement, description and prevention of oral disease and the promotion of oral health. It also refers to **art**. This involves advocacy, policy development and the politics of how dental care is prioritized, organized, monitored and paid for in societies.

The key components of dental public health practice and how these relate to one another are shown in Figure 1.1. The core values of public health practice are as in Table 1.1.

A comparison between clinical dental practice and dental public health practice is shown in Table 1.2.

The public health approach

The Faculty of Public Health, the professional body that is responsible for setting standards in public health practice in the UK, describes the public health approach as:
- population based

Table 1.1 Core values of public health practice as defined by the Faculty of Public Health in the UK

- Equitable
- Empowering
- Effective
- Evidence based
- Fair
- Inclusive

Table 1.2 A comparison between clinical dental practice and dental public health

Individual clinical practice	Public health practice
Individual patients	Populations and defined groups within populations
Examination	Epidemiology, surveys
Diagnosis	Assessment of need
Treatment planning	Prioritization and programme planning
Informed consent for treatment	Ethics and planning approval
An appropriate mix of care, cure and prevention	Programme implementation
Payment for services	Programme budgeting/finance
Evaluation	Appraisal and review

- emphasizing collective responsibility for health, its protection and disease prevention
- recognizing the key role of the state, linked to a concern for the underlying socio-economic and wider determinants of health, as well as disease
- emphasizing partnerships with all those who contribute to the health of the population.

How this applies to dental public health is shown in Table 1.3.

Key disciplines in dental public health

In order to practise dental public health, knowledge of the following disciplines is important.

Table 1.3 The public health approach as applied to dentistry

Dental public health:
- Is concerned with the oral health of populations
  - in a city or defined geographical area
  - in a particular group of the population defined by a common demographic, e.g. children, older people
  - in a group of people with social circumstances in common, e.g. homeless people, people with drug and substance abuse problems.
- Recognizes that responsibility for health and prevention of oral disease is shared between individual people and healthcare professionals, and that people should be empowered to look after their own health.
- Is conscious that as health is markedly linked to people's lifestyles and life circumstances, it needs to take account of how the risk of poor oral health is not equal across populations, e.g. levels of dental caries in children are closely correlated with social and economic deprivation.
- Implies that to improve health, it is necessary to work on policy development at a high level and across disciplines. As an example, legislation making the wearing of seat belts compulsory is important in preventing facial injuries in road traffic accidents; taxing tobacco sales is important in moderating smoking. In health improvement programmes in schools, dental public health practitioners need to work outside health and collaborate with school teachers and education authorities.

Oral epidemiology

Oral epidemiology is the study of oral health and oral disease and their determinants in populations.

Demography

This refers to measurements and statistics that describe populations. It involves recording factors such as the age structure of the population, ethnic composition and educational attainment.

Medical statistics

Understanding numbers and the inferences that can be drawn from them in reviewing disease trends and service provision is a key skill, as is the ability to appraise and conduct dental research.

Health promotion and health improvement

Health promotion is the process of enabling people to increase control over their health and its determinants and thereby to improve their health. Health improvement recognizes that the determinants of health can be outside an individual's control and is designed to address so-called *wider determinants of health* such as education, housing and employment. It is also designed to address the gaps in health between areas of high and low social and economic provision – gaps known as '*health inequalities*'.

Sociology

Sociology is the study of the development, structure and functioning of human societies. An understanding of these factors is important in improving health and organizing healthcare services.

Psychology

Psychology is the branch of science that deals with the human mind and its functions. In a public health context, an understanding of psychology is important in relation to behaviour change.

Health economics

Health economics concerns the need for, demand for and supply of health and healthcare. In the context of dental public health, it relates to how resources are distributed and the effectiveness and efficiency of services. How care is commissioned and paid for is an important element of how dentistry is organized and delivered, and dental public health practitioners need a clear understanding of these issues.

Health services management and planning

Dental services are in competition with other forms of healthcare, whether paid for by the state or by individuals. They therefore need to be organized, managed and planned. Allocation of resources within a publicly funded dental service should be done in proportion to need and likelihood of benefit. Dental public health practitioners will be called on to give advice to health service managers and finance officers on the appropriate allocation of resources and to offer guidance on how dental services are planned and delivered.

Evidence-based practice

Evidence-based practice is designed to ensure that wherever possible, the dental care that is delivered has been shown to be that which is most efficient and effective. It is the role of dental public health practitioners to facilitate such practice. Those responsible for dental public health need to understand the theory of evidence-based dentistry to support the improvement of oral health and the delivery of effective care.

2 Health, oral health and their determinants

Figure 2.1 The determinants of health. Source: *Adapted from Dahlgren and Whitehead (1991). Reproduced with permission from Institute for Futures Studies.*

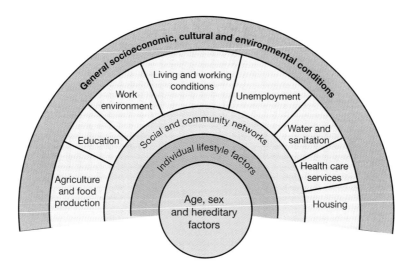

Figure 2.2 Life circumstances and lifestyle as determinants of health

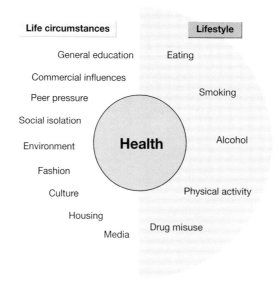

Figure 2.3 Lifecourse analysis as a means of investigating the determinants of health

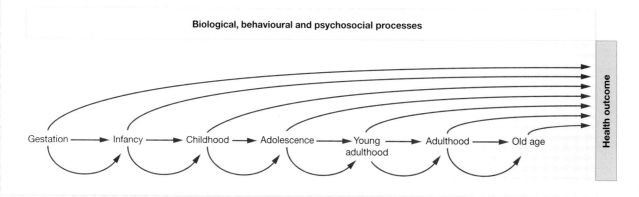

Dental Public Health at a Glance, First Edition. Ivor G. Chestnutt.
© 2016 John Wiley & Sons, Ltd. Published 2016 by John Wiley & Sons, Ltd.

Health

The most widely accepted definition of health is that offered by the World Health Organization in 1948, which states:

Health is a complete state of physical, mental and social wellbeing and not merely the absence of disease or infirmity.

The key point in this definition is that health is more than simply not being ill. It encompasses all of an individual's being. Today, health is also recognized as not solely a desired state to acquire, but a means to enable individuals to live their lives to the full and 'be all they can be'.

Oral health

Mirroring the definition of general health, oral health can be defined as follows:

Oral health is a standard of health of the oral and related tissues without active disease. That state should enable the individual to eat, speak and socialize without discomfort or embarrassment and contribute to general wellbeing.

This means that while a patient may have no active dental decay, or periodontal disease, if they are embarrassed by the appearance of their teeth when they smile, then they cannot be said to be have true oral health. This definition also recognizes that good oral health is integral to good overall health. Older people who cannot eat properly because they lack sufficient teeth or have inadequate dentures may become compromised nutritionally.

The impact of oral disease on individuals can be measured using **social-dental indicators** (Chapter 4).

Determinants of health and oral health

Determinant simply means 'factor influencing'. Many things can influence health. The diagram in Figure 2.1 was drawn by Dahlgren and Whitehead in 1991. It illustrates the concept of health being influenced by factors that operate at different levels.

Innate determinants of health

First, health is determined by factors innate to the individual. So age, gender and genetic make-up will all influence health. These determinants are not easily amenable to change. For example, a degree of attachment loss and periodontal recession is almost inevitable as a patient ages, although this will probably reflect a mixture of ageing and exposure to the next level of determinants, **lifestyle**.

Lifestyle as a determinant of health

Health and oral health can be markedly influenced by **lifestyle**. Diet, smoking, consumption of alcohol and lack of exercise all have the potential to influence health. Dental caries is caused by exposure to excess fermentable carbohydrates (sugars), and smoking tobacco is a significant risk factor in the aetiology of periodontal disease and oral cancer (Figure 2.2).

Life circumstances as determinants of health

While **lifestyle** can be thought of as things people do to themselves (behaviours), **life circumstances** are things that are done to people and are to a large degree outside their direct control. As an example, peer pressure may lead a teenager to feel compelled to have an intra-oral piercing, or advertising may persuade people to consume foods that are high in sugar (Figure 2.2).

Social and community networks as determinants of health

Interaction with others and the support that they provide are recognized as important determinants of health. Peer support and social interaction are necessary components of health for most people.

General socio-economic, cultural and environmental conditions as determinants of health

At the highest level, social and economic factors have a major influence on health. Policies decided at national and international levels have impacts on health. The ability of a community or country to provide basic education for its population, for example, will have an impact on health literacy. The proportion of a country's gross domestic product (GDP; i.e. the country's wealth) that is devoted to health services can influence how easy it is to access medical and dental care. There are large variations in the proportion of national wealth that is spent on health in different countries. In 2012 the United States spent 17.9% of GDP on healthcare, while the United Kingdom devoted 9.4% and France spent 11.7%. In developing countries the proportion of national wealth spent on health services is typically low, of the order of 3–5%, while at the same time vast sums are often spent on military and defence services.

The impact of the environment on health is of major concern. Worldwide issues such as global warming may in the long term have significant implications for health. However, even in the present environmental issues can influence health and oral health. Overexposure to sunshine and lack of use of protective sunscreens can cause skin cancers in the head and neck region. Underexposure to sunshine can result in lack of vitamin D and in diseases such as rickets.

Lifecourse analysis

This approach to understanding the determinants of health looks at how events in early life or across generations can affect susceptibility to disease in adulthood. Lifecourse studies investigate biological, psychological and behavioural factors and how these operate during gestation, childhood, adolescence and young adulthood to influence disease in later life (Figure 2.3). These types of study involve following up a cohort of people over time. An example is the Dunedin Multidisciplinary Health and Development study. This recruited a pool of children born in the Otago Region in New Zealand in 1972 and 1973 and has examined them at ages 3, 5, 7, 9, 11, 13, 15, 18, 21, 26, 32 and, most recently, at age 38 (2010–12). Oral health has been investigated as part of this study.

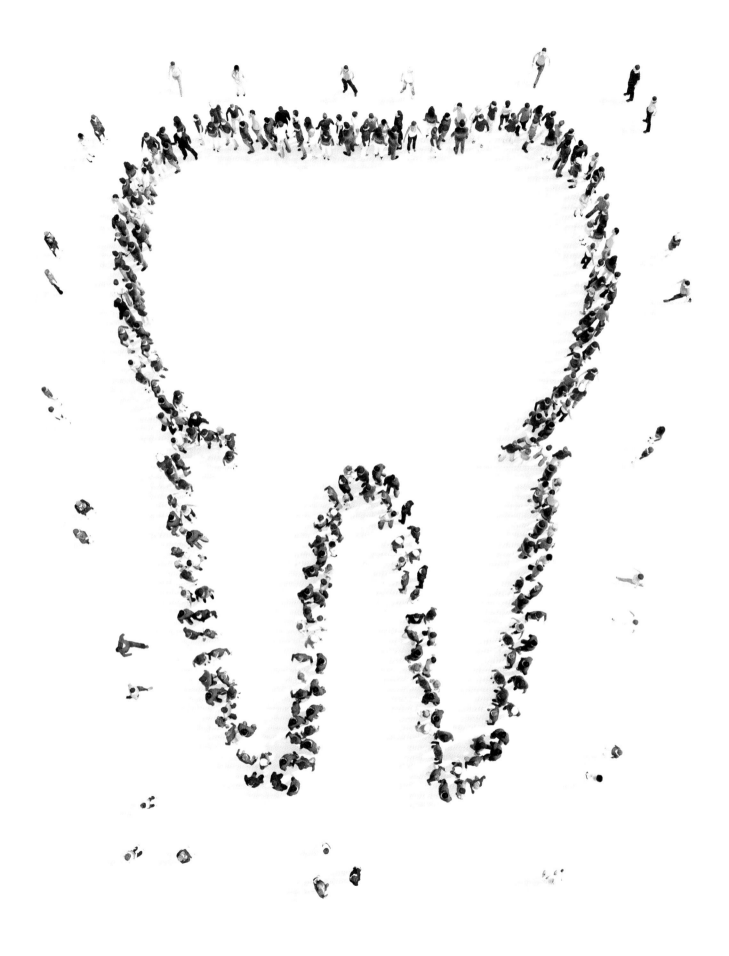

Epidemiology

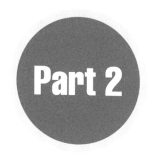

Part 2

Chapters

3 Basic epidemiology

Dental Public Health at a Glance, First Edition. Ivor G. Chestnutt.
© 2016 John Wiley & Sons, Ltd. Published 2016 by John Wiley & Sons, Ltd.

Figure 3.1   What is epidemiology?

Epidemiology is the study of the
distribution and determinants of
diseases and injuries in populations

– distribution = location
– determinant = cause or risk factor

Figure 3.2   The principle components of an epidemiological study

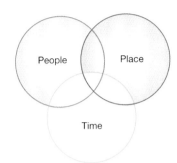

People   Place

Time

Figure 3.3   UK population by age and gender 2011 and 2001. Source: *Office for National Statistics 2012. Reproduced with permission from Office for National Statistics.*

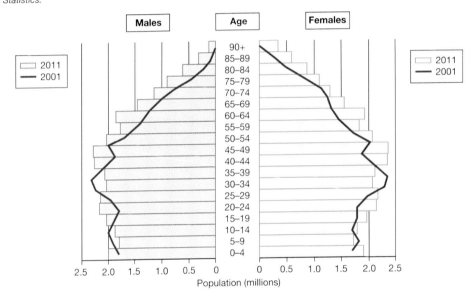

Epidemiology

Epidemiology, from 'epi' = about and 'demos' = people, is that branch of science that deals with the study of the distribution of health and illness and their determinants (or influencing factors) in populations or groups of people, at a particular time or over a period of time (Figure 3.1).

Thus, in an epidemiological study three key elements can be identified: people, place and time (Figure 3.2).

Describing disease in populations

Count data

The simplest measure in an epidemiological study is a count of the number of people in an area affected by a particular condition at one point in time. For example, it is possible to state that there were **x** people affected by oral cancer in a given country on a given day (assuming that we could accurately identify and count this). This information can be used to plan services. However, **count data** on their own are of limited value. This is because they do not contain **denominator data**. That means it is not known how many people have the condition out of those who could possibly be affected. So in the oral cancer example, simply reporting the number of people with oral cancer gives no idea of whether a large or small proportion of the population is affected. It would not therefore be possible to identify changes over time (as the number of people at risk may change) or to make comparisons between different areas or countries. For this reason, data in epidemiology are almost always reported as **rates** or **proportions**.

Prevalence

One of the most common ways of describing the amount of disease in a population is by reporting the *prevalence*.

*Prevalence is the proportion of people with a disease at any given point (**point prevalence**) or period (**period prevalence**) in time.*

Incidence

While prevalence describes the amount of disease present **at** a given point or period in time, incidence describes the amount of new disease that occurs **over** a given period of time.

Incidence is the number of new cases of a disease in a defined population over a defined period of time. Incidence measures events – a change from a healthy to a diseased state.

It is important to remember these terms and use them correctly. In common usage, for example in the press and media, the terms prevalence and incidence are frequently employed incorrectly and interchangeably without regard to their correct meaning.

Standardized data

Standardization is a technique that is used to account for the effect of confounding factors in populations.

Oral cancer is more common in older people and in men. If we are interested in deaths due to oral cancer, age and gender act as confounding factors. As a result, when comparing deaths from oral cancer between two cities, it is important to take into account the age and gender structure of those communities. For example, a city with a large student population would have a different age and gender structure to a seaside town to which many older people have retired.

Standardized mortality ratio (SMR)

To overcome this problem and allow comparison of deaths due to oral cancer, taking into account confounding factors, a **standardized mortality ratio** (SMR) is calculated:

$$\text{SMR} = \frac{\text{Observed number of deaths per year}}{\text{Expected number of deaths per year}} \times 100$$

To do this, the deaths in a particular area are compared with a wider population. In the above case we could calculate the deaths in different age bands and for males and females in the whole country. This constitutes the **expected** deaths. We could also work out the deaths in these same age bands and by gender in our university city or seaside town. This is the **observed** death rate. The actual or observed number of deaths can then be compared with the expected number. The ratio of observed to expected deaths gives the mortality ratio, and is usually expressed as a percentage. The mortality ratio in the whole county is 100 (because the number of expected and observed deaths is by definition the same). If the resulting value is greater than 100, that would indicate that oral cancer-related mortality was unfavourable, even having accounted for the age and gender structure of the population. A value of less than 100 indicates a more favourable mortality.

Demography

Demography is the scientific discipline that studies populations and how they are affected by factors such as births, deaths, gender, age structure and migration. Population structure can be represented by a **population pyramid**, such as that shown in Figure 3.3. The population is plotted in five-year age bands, with numbers of males on the left and numbers of females on the right. The shape can be used to deduce the relative number of old and young people in a population. The UK population structure is typical of a Western developed country, where the top of the pyramid is relatively broad, indicating a low young:old person ratio. A population pyramid for a developing country would have a much broader base and more steeply sloping sides, indicating a high young:old person ratio.

Increased longevity and a greater number of older people in the UK population have seen the ratio of young to old people decrease in recent years. Age structure can also be affected by migration. Migrants tend to be young and to have more children. Health service planners need to make provision for such population changes.

4 Principles of measuring and recording oral disease and oral health

Table 4.1 Common dental indices and the conditions they measure

Index	Condition measured
DMFT/dmft (decayed, missing and filled)	Dental caries
RCI (Root Caries Index)	Root caries
Community Periodontal Index of Treatment Need (CPITN) – Basic Periodontal Examination (BPE)	Periodontal disease
Plaque Index	Dental plaque
Modified Gingival Index	Gingivitis
IOTN (Index of Orthodontic Treatment Need)	Orthodontic treatment need
PAR (Peer Assessment Rating)	Orthodontic treatment outcome
Erosion Index	Erosion/non-carious tooth surface loss
Dean's Index	Fluorosis
Modified DDE	Developmental defects of enamel

Table 4.2 Interpretation of the strength of agreement determined by the kappa (κ) statistic

Value of κ	Strength of agreement
1.00–0.81	Very good
0.80–0.61	Good
0.60–0.41	Moderate
0.40–0.21	Fair
< 0.20	Poor

Table 4.3 Reasons for measuring and recording oral disease

At an INDIVIDUAL level	At a POPULATION level
Clinical management	
To aid diagnosis	To record the prevalence of disease in a population
To aid treatment	To aid understanding of the aetiology of diseases
To measure individual treatment need	To provide an indication of population treatment need
To measure individual treatment outcome	To evaluate the effectiveness of public health programmes
Research (e.g. in clinical trials)	
To test the effect of new treatments or products	

Table 4.4 Oral Health Impact Profile 14 (OHIP 14)

Dimension	Question – How often in the last 12 months…
Functional limitation	Have you had trouble *pronouncing any words* because of problems with your mouth, teeth or dentures?
	Have you felt that your *sense of taste* has worsened because of problems with your mouth, teeth or dentures?
Physical pain	Have you had *painful aching* in your mouth?
	Have you found it *uncomfortable to eat any foods* because of problems with your mouth, teeth or dentures?
Psychological discomfort	Have you been *self-conscious* because of your mouth, teeth or dentures?
	Have you *felt tense* because of problems with your mouth, teeth or dentures?
Physical disability	Has your *diet been unsatisfactory* because of problems with your mouth, teeth or dentures?
	Have you had to *interrupt meals* because of problems with your mouth, teeth or dentures?
Psychological disability	Have you found it *difficult to relax* because of problems with your mouth, teeth or dentures?
	Have you been a bit *embarrassed* because of problems with your mouth, teeth or dentures?
Social disability	Have you been a bit *irritable with other people* because of problems with your mouth, teeth or dentures?
	Have you had *difficulty doing your usual jobs* because of problems with your mouth, teeth or dentures?
Handicap	Have you felt that life in general was *less satisfying* because of problems with your mouth, teeth or dentures?
	Have you been *totally unable to function* because of problems with your mouth, teeth or dentures?

Responses on a 5-point scale coded 0=never, 1=hardly ever, 2=occasionally, 3=fairly often, 4=very often

Source: *Slade 1997. Reproduced with permission from John Wiley & Sons.*

Dental Public Health at a Glance, First Edition. Ivor G. Chestnutt.
© 2016 John Wiley & Sons, Ltd. Published 2016 by John Wiley & Sons, Ltd.

What is a dental index?

In order to record the presence of dental disease, a suitable means of recording the presence, extent and severity of the condition, in a consistent fashion, is required. Such recording systems are termed **dental indices** (singular dental index). Over the years, numerous dental indices have been developed and standardized ways of recording most dental conditions and pathologies exist. Examples of commonly used dental indices are shown in Table 4.1.

The properties of an ideal dental index

An ideal dental index should have the following features:
• **Simple** – The index should be simple to understand and easy to learn. This is important if large numbers of clinicians are to be taught how to use the index in a consistent fashion. It should also be simple to administer. An index that takes a long time to record reduces the efficiency of collecting data in epidemiological surveys, where clinicians need to record a large amount of data in a short period of time.
• **Objective** – There should be as little scope as possible for subjective interpretation on the part of the examining clinician. This limits the chances of different clinicians recording different levels of disease when examining identical clinical conditions.
• **Clear-cut categories** – The division between different categories or codes used within an index should be clear. It is also helpful if these categories relate to distinct stages of the clinical condition being measured. If these distinct stages relate to different treatment needs, then it is possible to construct an index that not only measures the presence of a disease, but can give an **indication of treatment need**. Common examples include the Community Periodontal Index of Treatment Need (CPITN) and the Index of Orthodontic Treatment Need (IOTN).
• **Valid** – The index must measure what it is intended to measure. For example, an index designed to measure early dental decay (white spots) must not be confused by developmental hypoplasia (which can also appear as a white/demineralized spot).
• **Reliable** – Each time the index is used it should record the same outcome (provided of course that the disease remains the same). This relates to the properties of the index.
• **Reproducible** – Each time the index is used it should record the same outcome, either when two different examiners use the index to measure the same condition (**inter-examiner reproducibility**) or when the same examiner measures the condition on two different occasions (**intra-examiner reproducibility**). This is provided, of course, that the condition being measured has not changed between examinations. The degree of agreement between or within examiners is measured statistically using the **Kappa statistic (κ)**. This is a more robust measure than simply calculating the percentage agreement between examiners, as κ takes into account agreement that has occurred by chance. The Kappa statistic is reported as a value between 0 and 1 and it is interpreted as shown in Table 4.2.
• **Quantifiable** – It is an advantage if the output of a dental index is amenable to statistical analysis.
• **Sensitive** – An ideal index should be able to detect and record small changes in levels of disease.
• **Reversible** – A good index should respond to improvements in the dental condition being measured.
• **Future risk** – It is an advantage if a dental index can give an indication of the future risk of disease.
Few dental indices meet all of these ideal characteristics.

Why is it necessary to measure and record dental disease?

Measuring dental diseases can be viewed from two perspectives: in the context of measuring disease either in an **individual in a clinical context**, or in an **individual as part of a population group**. The reasons for measuring in these contexts are described in Table 4.3.

Many dental indices were initially developed for use in research studies (e.g. plaque and gingivitis indices) and then subsequently used in clinical treatment settings. Other indices employed in the diagnosis and clinical management of patients were derived from indices initially developed for use in epidemiological surveys. For instance, the Basic Periodontal Examination (BPE) evolved from the Community Periodontal Index of Treatment Need (CPITN).

Socio-dental indicators of oral health

The dental indicators described in Table 4.1 measure dental diseases from a **normative** perspective. That means that the disease is very much judged from a clinician's perspective. Therefore these indices do not capture the full impact of the disease on the patient in terms of how they function, or the impact of the disease on their general health or on their lifestyle and daily living. A range of indices called **socio-dental indicators** have been developed to capture the impact of dental and oral disease beyond the mainly physical signs and symptoms on which traditional indices rely.

A commonly used socio-dental indicator is the **Oral Health Impact Profile (OHIP)**. When originally devised this comprised 49 questions, but a more user-friendly version with just 14 questions has been developed (**OHIP-14**; see Table 4.4). This asks two questions on each of seven dimensions of impact. Patients are asked using a five-point scale how commonly they have experienced these impacts in the past 12 months and a score is derived. This can be used to compare the impact with population norms or to investigate the effect of providing different forms of treatment.

5 Epidemiology of dental caries

Figure 5.1 The DMF/dmf index for recording dental caries

D/d = decay M/m = missing F/f = filled

DMF – refers to the *permanent* dentition

dmf – refers to the *primary* dentition

DMFT – refers to teeth and indicates the number of permanent teeth, filled, missing or decayed. Can score 0–32 (0–28 if exclude 3rd molars).

dmft indicates the number of primary teeth, filled, missing or decayed. Can score 0–20

DMFS – refers to the number of surfaces of permanent teeth filled, missing or decayed. If missing due to caries: Incisors and canines count as 4 surfaces, premolars and molars as 5.

DMFS can score 0–148 (0–128 if exclude 3rd molars)

dmfs can score 0–88

Components of DMF can be used to determine:

$\dfrac{D}{DMF}$ = index of treatment need

$\dfrac{F}{DMF}$ = Index of treatment provision (or Care Index)

$\dfrac{M}{DMF}$ = Index of treatment failure

Figure 5.2 Extent of dental decay as defined in conventional dental epidemiology surveys

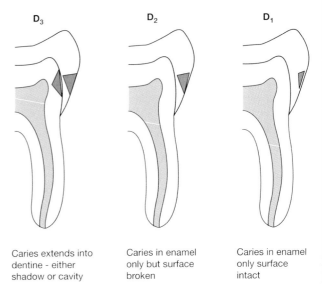

D_3	D_2	D_1
Caries extends into dentine - either shadow or cavity	Caries in enamel only but surface broken	Caries in enamel only surface intact

Figure 5.3 Calculation of the significant caries index.
Source: *Adapted from Bratthall 2000 with permission from John Wiley & Sons.*

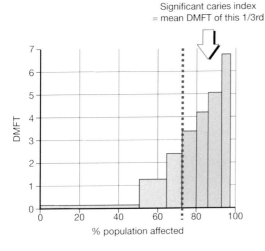

Figure 5.4 Obvious dental decay in 15 year olds in the UK 1973–2013. Source: *Health and Social Care Information Centre 2015. (1973 = England & Wales only, 2014 = England, Wales and Northern Ireland)*

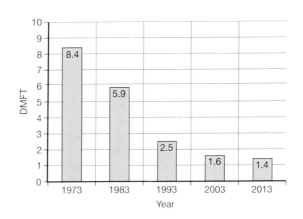

Figure 5.5 Schematic representation of changes in the distribution of dental caries in children in the United Kingdom 1970 and 2015

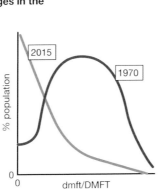

Dental Public Health at a Glance, First Edition. Ivor G. Chestnutt.

Recording dental caries in oral health surveys

The DMF/dmf Index

Dental caries is recorded using the DMF/dmf Index. This records the number of teeth that are **d**ecayed, **m**issing or **f**illed as a result of dental caries (DMFT/dmft) or the number of tooth surfaces (DMFS/dmfs) similarly affected. Conventions for use of the index are shown in Figure 5.1.

This is the most widely used caries index. Decay can be scored at the D_1, D_2 and D_3 levels (Figure 5.2). The majority of dental surveys and clinical trials around the world have been conducted using the DMF Index, with caries scored at the D_3 level, or into dentine (Figure 5.2). The components of the index can be used to calculate treatment need, provision and failure.

ICDAS International Caries Detection and Assessment System

This index uses two scores per tooth surface. The first code relates to the restorative status of the tooth, the second to the caries status. The ICDAS index was developed primarily to enable the degree of caries progress into dental enamel to be recorded in greater detail than is possible with the traditional DMF Index. Full details of the index can be found on the ICDAS website (www.icdas.org).

Significant Caries Index

This index was developed to take account of the skewed distribution of dental caries in populations. The large proportion of caries-free individuals can mask the true extent of caries in affected individuals by reducing the population mean (Figure 5.3). To calculate the Significant Caries Index, individuals are sorted according to their DMFT values. The third of the population with the highest caries score is selected and the mean DMFT for this subgroup is calculated.

Epidemiological surveys for dental caries

There is a long history of oral health surveys in the United Kingdom.

Decennial surveys

Since 1968 a series of surveys of the oral health of adults and children has been conducted every ten years (traditionally adults in years ending in 8, although the 2008 survey slipped to 2009, and children in years ending in 3). These initially covered all of the United Kingdom, but following devolution of responsibility for health to the Scottish Parliament, Scotland has not participated in the most recent surveys, instead having instituted its own dental inspection programme as a means of surveying oral health in children.

BASCD surveys

In addition to the decennial surveys, a long-standing series of surveys of children's oral health has been conducted across the United Kingdom by local health bodies in collaboration with the British Association for the Study of Community Dentistry. The decennial and BASCD surveys have provided key information for oral health needs assessment and dental service planning.

Caries prevalence in the United Kingdom

Children

Figure 5.4 shows changes in the prevalence of dental caries in 15-year-olds. This illustrates the remarkable improvement that there has been in oral health in the United Kingdom in the past four decades. It is difficult for the current generation of dental students to appreciate a time when half of all 15-year-olds had eight or more decayed permanent teeth. The changes observed can to a large part be attributed to the introduction of fluoride-containing toothpaste, which became widely available from the early 1970s onwards.

Adults

The number of sound untreated teeth by age in England is shown in Table 5.1. From this it is apparent that mean number of teeth unaffected by dental caries increased across all age groups between 1978 and 2009. Changes in the pattern of tooth loss in adults are shown in Figure 9.1.

Changes in the distribution of dental caries in the population

An important change in the way dental caries is distributed across the population occurred as oral health improved. In the early 1970s, dental caries in children was normally distributed; that is, while a small number of the population were caries free, the majority of the population experienced decay to a greater or lesser degree. As oral health improved, the caries-free proportion of the population increased, but the disease burden fell on a smaller proportion of the population. The distribution of the disease became skewed (Figure 5.5). Those affected by caries increasingly were from more deprived social and economic circumstances (see Chapter 19). This gives rise to the concept of a 'high-risk' group in the population.

Table 5.1 Mean number of sound and untreated teeth by age in England, 1978–2009

Age (years)	1978	1988	1998	2009
16–24	17.5	21.7	23.7	26.1
25–34	14.1	16.4	19.5	24.0
35–44	12.4	13.3	15.9	20.4
45–54	10.6	11.7	11.9	15.2
55–64	9.2	9.5	9.7	12.0
65+			8.6	9.6
All	13.2	15.0	15.6	18.0

Source: *Data from Health and Social Care Information Centre (2011). N.B. The criteria changed after 1998.*

6 Epidemiology of periodontal disease

Figure 6.1 Common plaque and gingival indices. Source: *Data from Greene and Vermillion 1960; from Silness and Löe 1964; and from Löe 1967.*

Debris index (DI)	Silness & Löe 1964	Löe 1967

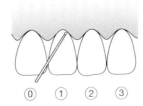

**Debris index
(Greene & Vermillion 1960)**

0 = No plaque

1 = Plaque covering 1/3 tooth

2 = Plaque covering 2/3 tooth

3 = Plaque totally covering tooth

**Plaque index
(Silness & Löe 1964)**

0 = No plaque detected

1 = Looks clean but material can be removed from gingival third with probe

2 = Visible plaque

3 = Tooth covered with abundant plaque

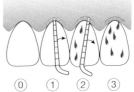

**Modified gingival index
(Löe 1967)**

0 = Healthy gingivae

1 = Gingivae look inflamed, but don't bleed when probed

2 = Gingivae look inflamed and bleed when probed

3 = Ulceration and spontaneous bleeding

Figure 6.2 Community Periodontal Index Treatment Need probe

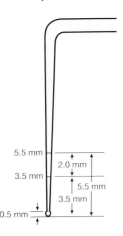

Figure 6.3 Susceptibility to periodontitis

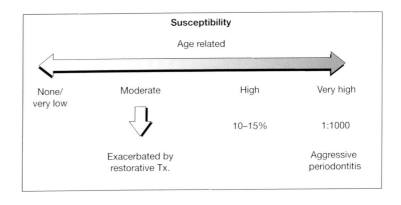

Figure 6.4 Periodontal health by age group, UK 2009. Source: *Data from Health and Social Care Information Centre 2011.*

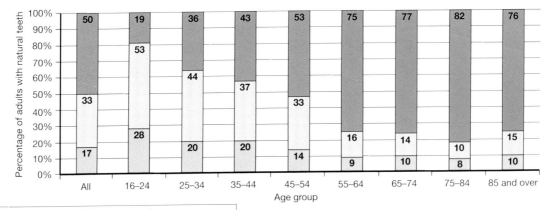

Periodontal disease includes all pathological conditions of the periodontium, but commonly refers to inflammatory conditions that are induced by dental plaque – namely, **gingivitis** and **periodontitis**. Gingivitis is an inflammatory response of the gingivae without destruction of the tooth-supporting apparatus. Periodontitis results in destruction of the fibres and bone that support the tooth and initially presents as the development of a periodontal pocket.

Periodontal indices

In measuring the prevalence of periodontal disease, the primary clinical features that are recorded are the presence and amount of dental plaque and calculus, inflammation of the gingivae, presence and depth of periodontal pockets, attachment loss (pocket depth plus recession) and mobility of teeth. Numerous periodontal indices have been developed to measure these features (Figure 6.1). The Community Periodontal Index of Treatment Need (CPITN) was developed by the World Health Organization. A specially designed probe is used to measure pocket depth (Figure 6.2). The mouth is divided into sextants (two posterior and one anterior per arch) and the worst score per sextant is recorded (Table 6.1).

Susceptibility to periodontitis

The prevalence of periodontal pocketing increases with age, but severe periodontitis affects only 10–15% of the population. The prevalence of severe periodontitis worldwide is reported in Table 10.1. A much smaller proportion of the population (about 1 in 1000) is affected by aggressive periodontitis, which results in severe loss of alveolar bone and deep periodontal pockets at a young age (Figure 6.3).

Periodontal health in the United Kingdom

The periodontal status of those with natural teeth in the 2009 UK Adult Dental Health Survey is shown in Figure 6.4. The authors of that survey reported periodontal status as:
• Periodontally healthy: defined as no bleeding, no calculus, no pocketing or loss of attachment greater than 4 mm.
• Periodontally healthy but with calculus or bleeding, no pockets or loss of attachment greater than 4 mm.
• Some periodontal disease present – pocketing of 4 mm or more present.
Overall just 17% of adults were deemed to be totally periodontally healthy; that is, no pockets > 4 mm and no bleeding or calculus.

The prevalence of periodontal disease increased with age, such that from age 55 and over, at least 75% of the population had a periodontal pocket or attachment loss of at least 4 mm at one or more sites.

While the prevalence of periodontal pockets increases with age, only a small proportion of the population experiences periodontal disease at a level that will cause them to lose a large number of teeth.

Oral cleanliness and oral hygiene practices

In the 2009 UK Adult Dental Health Survey, two-thirds (66%) of adults had dental plaque present on at least one tooth and there were on average six teeth on which plaque deposits could be detected. A similar proportion (68%) had calculus present in at least one sextant of their mouths.

In this survey, 75% of adults claimed to brush their teeth twice per day. Women were more likely to do so than men (82% vs 67%). A further 23% of the population claimed to brush their teeth once a day. Only 2% reported brushing less than once per day and 1% suggested that they never brushed their teeth at all.

An association was observed between frequency of tooth brushing and socioeconomic status. While 79% of adults from managerial and professional backgrounds said they brushed their teeth twice a day, in routine and manual occupation households the corresponding figure was 68%.

The use of other products to clean teeth was reported by 58% of dentate adults, with mouthwash (31%), electric toothbrushes (26%) and dental floss (21%) being the most frequently cited.

Risk factors for periodontal disease

Individuals are not equally at risk of developing periodontal disease. A longitudinal study of periodontal disease in New York State identified the risk factors and associated odds ratios as shown in Table 6.2.

Periodontal disease and systemic disease

In the past decade a great deal of research effort has been expended on determining the possible effect of periodontal disease on general health. The two systemic conditions that have received most attention are cardiovascular disease and pre-term low-birthweight babies. The results of these studies are often contradictory and the true nature of the impact of periodontal disease on general health awaits determination.

Table 6.1 CPITN scores

CPITN score	Clinical parameters
Code 0	Healthy, no pockets > 3.5 mm, no bleeding on probing, no calculus, no defective restoration margins
Code 1	No pockets > 3.5 mm, bleeding on probing but no calculus, no defective restoration margins
Code 2	No pockets > 3.5 mm, bleeding on probing and either calculus or defective restoration margins
Code 3	Pockets > 3.5 mm < 5.5 mm
Code 4	Pockets > 5.5 mm

Table 6.2 Odds ratio associated with various risk factors for periodontal attachment loss

Variable	Estimated odds ratio
Age	1.72–9.01
Smoking	2.05–4.75
Diabetes	2.32
P gingivalis	1.59
Education	0.65

Source: *Data from Grossi et al. 1994.*

7 Epidemiology of oral cancer

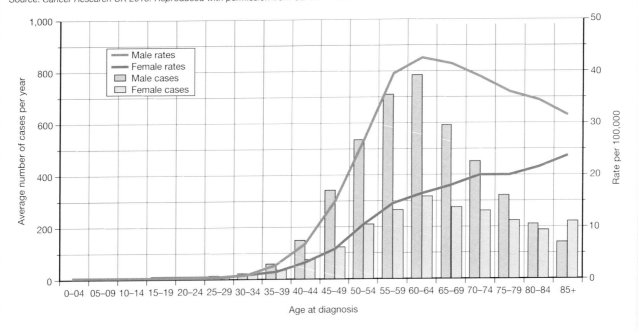

Figure 7.1 Average number of new cases per year and age-specific incidence rates per 100,000 population, UK, 2009–2011.
Source: *Cancer Research UK 2015. Reproduced with permission from Cancer Research UK.*

Table 7.3 Risk factors for oral cancer

Risk factor	Notes
Smoking tobacco	Oral cancer is three times more common in smokers compared with those who have never smoked.
Smokeless tobacco	Increases the risk of oral cancer between 2 and 7 times.
Betel quid (a combination of betel leaf, areca nut and slaked lime)	Quid increases the risk of oral cancer by 3.5 (used without tobacco) and 7 times (used with tobacco). Use of betel (a type of nut with stimulant properties) is widespread in the Asia and Pacific region and is responsible for the high incidence of oral cancer in those areas. Immigrants from those areas may continue the practice in the United Kingdom, e.g. Bangladeshi women.
Alcohol	Consumption of alcohol increases the risk of oral cancer. It has been calculated that risk increases by 35% in men and 9% in women for every 1.5 units of alcohol consumed per day.
Human papilloma virus (HPV)	HPV, particularly strain 16, is associated with oral cancer and increasingly accepted as a risk factor. Transmission is by oral sex. An estimated 8% of oral cavity cancers and 14% of oropharyngeal cancers in the United Kingdom are linked to HPV infection.
Family history	Head and neck cancer risk is 70% higher in people with a family (particularly sibling) history of head and neck cancer, versus those without such a history.
Socio-economic status (SES)	There is evidence that oral cancer is associated with SES, even when other risk factors such as tobacco and alcohol have been controlled for.
Diet	Malnutrition is particularly associated with excess alcohol consumption and smoking. There is some suggestion that consumption of a diet rich in fruits and vegetables, and therefore in antioxidants, is protective against oral cancer.

Data sources for oral cancer

Assimilating data on oral cancer can be difficult, as each different anatomical site such as the tongue, lips and oropharynx is given a specific code. The International Classification of Diseases (ICD) codes oral cancer as ICD-10 C00-C06, C09-C10 and C12-C14 (which include the lip, tongue, mouth, oropharynx, piriform sinus, hypopharynx and other ill-defined sites of the lip, oral cavity and pharynx). In the United Kingdom, Cancer Registries in each of the constituent countries record all new cases and mortality due to oral cancer. These data are very usefully combined and presented for the United Kingdom by Cancer Research UK (www .cancerresearchuk.org).

The incidence of oral cancer – United Kingdom

In the United Kingdom oral cancer accounts for about 2% of all cancers and is the 12th most common cancer in males and 16th most common cancer in females. In 2011 there were 6767 new cases of oral cancer in the UK, 4510 (67%) in males and 2257 in females (Table 7.1). In 2010 the lifetime risk for developing oral cancer was 1 in 84 for men and 1 in 160 for women. The distribution of oropharyngeal cancer by anatomical site is shown in Table 7.2.

Geographical variation

The incidence of oral cancer (when adjusted to take account of different age structures in the populations of the individual countries – European Age Standardised) varies across the United Kingdom. The incidence in males in Scotland is 16.6 per 100,000 compared to 12.3 in England. This likely reflects differences in consumption of alcohol and use of tobacco.

Impact of age

Like most cancers, oral cancer is more common in older people. In males, 15% of cases were diagnosed in those aged 75 and older, the vast majority (71%) being diagnosed in those aged 50–74 years. The age at which cancer is diagnosed in women differs: 29% are aged 75 or more when first diagnosed, 59% being in the 50–74 year age group (Figure 7.1).

Table 7.1 Number of new cases of oral cancer in the UK and its constituent countries in 2011, as crude number of cases and European age-standardized incidence rate per 100,000 population

	Measure	England	Wales	Scotland	Northern Ireland	United Kingdom
Male	Number of cases	3609	275	504	122	4510
	Age-adjusted rate	12.3	15.3	16.6	12.7	12.8
Female	Number of cases	1810	108	270	69	2257
	Age-adjusted rate	5.2	5.1	7.5	6.2	5.4
Persons	Number of cases	5419	383	774	191	6767
	Age-adjusted rate	8.6	10.1	11.8	9.3	9.0

Source: *Cancer Research UK 2015. Reproduced with permission from Cancer Research UK.*

Table 7.2 Number of new cases of oral and oropharyngeal cancer in the UK in 2010 by anatomical site and the male-to-female ratio

Anatomical site (ICD-10 Code)	Number of new cases N	Number of new cases %	Male: Female ratio
Lip (C00)	381	5.8	1.9
Tongue (C01-C02)	2028	31.0	1.9
Mouth (C03-C06)	1920	29.4	1.3
Oropharynx (C09-C10)	1456	22.3	2.7
Piriform sinus (C12)	285	4.4	4.3
Hypopharynx (C13)	209	3.2	2.3
Other and ill-defined sites (C14)	260	4.0	2.3

Source: *Cancer Research UK 2015. Reproduced with permission from Cancer Research UK.*

Impact of socio-economic status (SES)

The chance of developing oral cancer is greater for those from low social and economic status. A systematic review and meta-analysis of case-control studies from around the world reported that when compared with individuals from high SES, those with a low occupation-related social class were 2.4 times more likely to develop oral cancer.

Trends

The incidence of oral cancer has increased markedly since the mid-1970s. When adjusted to account for differences in the age structure of the population across the years, the incidence of oral cancer has increased by 88% in men and 82% in women.

There is also evidence of an increased number of relatively young people presenting with oral cancer – people who lack the traditional risk factors of alcohol and tobacco. In these cases it is believed that infection with human papilloma virus (HPV), acquired by sexual activity, is likely to play an important role.

Mortality

There were 2119 deaths from oral cancer in the United Kingdom in 2012.

Survival

Overall about 40 men and 43 women in every 100 diagnosed with oral and oropharyngeal cancer will still be alive five years after initial diagnosis, but this rises to 90 in 100 in the case of lip cancer. The outcome is influenced by the stage of cancer at diagnosis. Early diagnosis is associated with lesser morbidity and mortality.

The incidence of oral cancer – international

The incidence of oral cancer varies around the world. In Europe oral cancer accounts for about 2% of all cancers, similar to the United Kingdom. It is highest in Hungary and lowest in Greece. In the United States oral cancer also accounts for about 2–3% of all cancers. The area where the incidence of oral cancer is greatest is Asia. In south central Asia, cancer of the oral cavity ranks among the three most common types of cancer.

Risk factors for oral cancer

Risk factors for oral cancer are largely attributable to lifestyle factors and are summarized in Table 7.3.

8 Epidemiology of malocclusion, non-carious tooth surface loss and traumatic dental injuries

Figure 8.1 **The percentage of adults in the UK with any, moderate or severe tooth wear.** Source: *Data from Health and Social Care Information Centre 2011.*

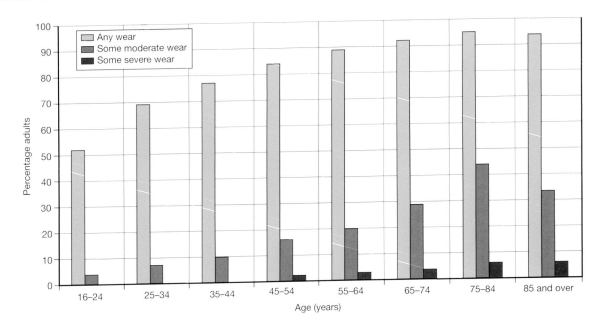

Table 8.1 Orthodontic condition of 12- and 15-year-old children by gender in the UK, 2003

	12 years			15 years		
	Boys	Girls	All	Boys	Girls	All
	Percentage of children					
Children undergoing orthodontic treatment at the time of the survey	7	10	8	12	16	14
Children not undergoing orthodontic treatment at the time of the survey						
Definite need for orthodontic treatment (DHC 4–5 and/or AC 8–10)	35	36	35	24	19	21
No definite need for orthodontic treatment (DHC 1–3 and AC 1–7)	58	55	57	64	65	65

Source: *Data from Health and Social Care Information Centre 2011.*

Table 8.2 Percentage of children aged 8, 12 and 15 years in the UK who experienced tooth surface loss (TSL) in permanent incisors and first permanent molars, 2003

	Age					
	8		12		15	
Year	1993[a]	2003	1993	2003	1993	2003
	Percentage of children					
INCISORS						
Buccal surfaces						
Any TSL	4	4	9	12	12	14
TSL into dentine or pulp	0	0	0	0	0	0
Lingual surfaces						
Any TSL	11	14	27	30	27	33
TSL into dentine or pulp	0	1	1	3	2	5
MOLARS						
Occlusal surface						
Any TSL		10		19		22
TSL into dentine or pulp		0		2		4

[a]TSL affecting first permanent molars was not measured in 1993.

Source: *Data from Health and Social Care Information Centre 2011.*

Malocclusion

Malocclusion describes the situation where the interdigitation and alignment of the teeth and jaws are less than ideal. This occurs due to misalignment of the teeth, or a discrepancy in the underlying relationship of the skeletal base or a combination of both. Clinically, malocclusion is measured using the **Index of Orthodontic Treatment Need (IOTN)**. The index has two parts: a Dental Health Component (DHC) and an Aesthetic Component (AC). The DHC is graded 1–5, where 1 = no treatment need and 5 = definite treatment need. The AC comprises a series of 10 intraoral clinical photographs in which the attractiveness of the teeth decreases from 1 to 10. The measurements required to undertake a full IOTN assessment are too time consuming for application in epidemiological surveys and so a modified version of the IOTN has been developed – this uses a simpler DHC plus the original AC.

The **modified version of the IOTN** examines five aspects of the dentition, Missing teeth, Overjet, Crossbites, Displacement of contact points (crowding) and Overbite, remembered using the acronym MOCDO:

M – Missing Teeth	Hypodontia requiring pre-restorative orthodontics or orthodontic space closure to obviate the need for a prosthesis
	Impeded eruption of teeth
	Presence of supernumerary teeth
	Retained deciduous teeth
O – Overjet	Increased overjet greater than 6 mm
	Reverse overjet greater than 3.5 mm with no masticatory or speech difficulties
	Reverse overjet greater than 1 mm but less than 3.5 mm with recorded masticatory and speech difficulties
C – Crossbites	Anterior or posterior crossbites with greater than 2 mm discrepancy between retruded contact position and intercuspal position
D – Displacement of contact points (crowding)	Contact point displacements greater than 4 mm
O – Overbite	Lateral or anterior open bites greater than 4 mm
	Deep overbite with gingival or palatal trauma

If any one of the above occlusal anomalies is present, the subject is said to have a definite need for orthodontic treatment (Source: Adapted from Burden et al. 2001).

The orthodontic condition of 12- and 15-year-old children in the United Kingdom as recorded in the 2003 Dental Health Survey of Children and Young People is shown in Table 8.1.

Qualification for treatment by the National Health Service

In the United Kingdom, the IOTN is used to determine whether a patient's malocclusion is sufficiently severe to merit treatment by the National Health Service. To qualify the DHC must be 3 or greater or the AC must be 6 or greater.

Non-carious tooth surface loss (tooth wear)

Tooth surface loss (TSL) can result from erosion, attrition or abrasion. Erosion results from the action of acidic foods and drinks (e.g. carbonated beverages) or the acidic contents of the stomach after repeated vomiting (as occurs in some eating disorders) or gastric regurgitation. Attrition results from the contact of teeth with the opposing dentition, and abrasion from the contact of teeth with external objects placed in the mouth, such as hard toothbrushes and abrasive toothpaste.

Tooth surface loss in children

A degree of attrition in the primary dentition is normal. However, exposure to a diet high in acidic foods and especially carbonated drinks has resulted in concerns over the degree of tooth wear in teenagers. In the 2003 Dental Health Survey of Children and Young People, tooth surface loss (TSL) was measured on the upper incisors and on molar teeth. The prevalence of TSL by age and degree (recorded as any TSL and TSL into dentine or pulp) is shown in Table 8.2.

Tooth surface loss in adults

Tooth wear was also measured in the 2009 Adult Dental Health Survey. In those adults with teeth, 77% showed some degree of tooth wear, 15% had moderate wear and 2% exhibited severe tooth loss. As would be expected, tooth wear and the severity of tooth wear increased with age, as shown in Figure 8.1. A greater proportion of males (82%) experienced tooth wear than did females (73%).

Traumatic dental injuries

Accidental injury to children's teeth is common. The frequency of injury is greater in boys, in children with an increased overjet and in children from households from a lower social and economic class.

The proportion of children who had experienced accidental damage to their teeth in the United Kingdom is shown in Table 8.3.

Prevention of traumatic dental injuries

Prevention of traumatic dental injuries has largely focused on the provision of mouthguards when participating in contact sports. While intuitively this seems a sensible measure, the degree to which mouthguards prevent dental injury has yet to be definitively established. The main limitation of this approach is that the majority of traumatic dental injuries do not occur when participating in organized sports but as a result of accidents during normal play and during slips, trips and falls. Dental injuries as a result of cycling, skateboarding and riding scooters are also regularly encountered in emergency dental clinics. Preventive strategies need to focus on increasing public awareness of dental injuries and in particular what to do in the event of an injury.

Table 8.3 Percentage of children aged 8, 12 and 15 years in the UK who had experienced accidental damage to their permanent dentition by gender and age, 2003

Year	1983	1993	2003
Gender/age	*Percentage of children*		
Boys			
8	12	6	6
12	29	25	14
15	33	21	16
Girls			
8	7	5	4
12	16	9	8
15	19	12	10
All children			
8	10	6	5
12	23	17	11
15	26	17	13

Source: *Data from Health and Social Care Information Centre 2011.*

National trends in oral health

Figure 9.1 Loss of all natural teeth by age in UK 1968–2009. Source: *Data from Health and Social Care Information Centre 2011.*
(2009 = England, Wales & N Ireland only)

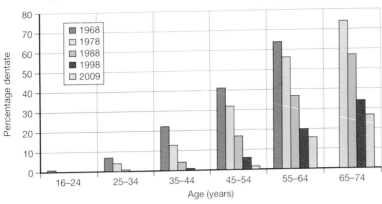

Figure 9.2 Time series and future projection of adult oral health in the UK 1998–2030. Source: *NHS England Dental Analytical Team 2014.*

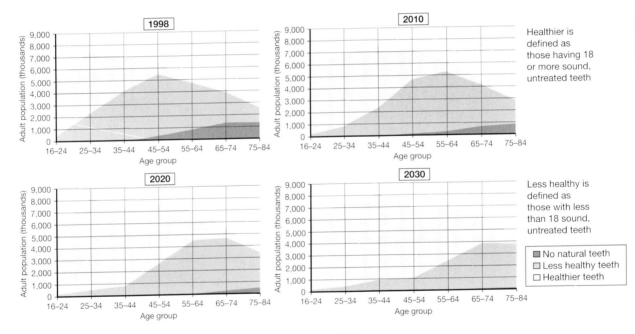

Healthier is defined as those having 18 or more sound, untreated teeth

Less healthy is defined as those with less than 18 sound, untreated teeth

- No natural teeth
- Less healthy teeth
- Healthier teeth

Figure 9.3 A schematic of the changing picture of oral health in the UK

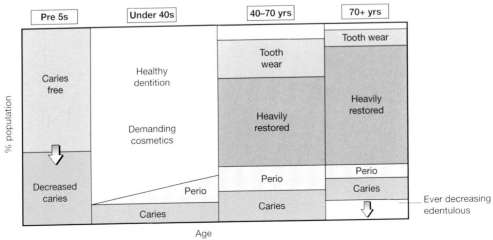

Dental Public Health at a Glance, First Edition. Ivor G. Chestnutt.
© 2016 John Wiley & Sons, Ltd. Published 2016 by John Wiley & Sons, Ltd.

The decennial adult oral health surveys (Chapter 5) provide data that show how oral health has changed in the past four decades. It is possible to model how these changes will be carried forward in time and from that to infer how future oral health and oral care needs will change.

Changes in oral health

Decrease in tooth loss

The most remarkable change in oral health over the last century has been a dramatic reduction in the proportion of the adult population who have had all of their teeth extracted. In the mid-twentieth century it was common for people in the United Kingdom to have all of their teeth extracted in early adulthood. This procedure was known as a 'dental clearance'. In the 1968 Adult Dental Health Survey, edentulous patients (i.e. those who had had all of their teeth extracted) were asked how many teeth were removed at the time they were rendered edentulous. In response, two-thirds said that they had had 12 or more teeth removed and one third had had 21 or more teeth removed – a scenario that is difficult to imagine today. Tooth removal was often carried out under general anaesthesia in dental practices. This reflected attitudes to oral health at that time, where removal of teeth and provision of complete dentures were often the only solution to the high levels of dental caries then prevalent.

Since the late 1960s the proportion of the population who have lost all of their own teeth has fallen dramatically (Figure 9.1) and overall the proportion of the UK population who are edentulous has fallen from 30% in 1978 to 6% in 2009.

Increase in sound and untreated teeth

Figure 9.2 shows estimates of how the proportion of the population with 18 or more sound untreated teeth will increase in the next two decades.

Changes in oral health across the generations

A schematic picture of what is happening to oral health across the generations is shown in Figure 9.3. While dental caries remains a problem in children from disadvantaged backgrounds (Chapter 19), oral health in children and young adults has improved dramatically (Figure 5.4).

A key factor in the improvement in oral health in the United Kingdom has been the introduction of fluoride-containing toothpaste. Fluoride toothpaste has been widely available since the early 1970s and is the factor that is often quoted as the key determinant of improved oral health in the last half-century.

People in middle to early older age, born prior to the general availability of fluoride toothpaste, often have retained the majority of their teeth because they have been able to take advantage of the increased availability and technical capability of dental services. Many of their teeth are heavily restored and will require continuing maintenance into old age. This segment of the population has been referred to as the '**heavy metal generation**', – perhaps reflecting their musical tastes, but also the fact that their dentition is largely composed of metal restorations.

The proportion of older people who are edentulous will decrease over time, so that by 2030 the proportion of the population who will have lost all of their teeth will be very small (Figure 9.2).

Reasons for improved oral health

The following are the likely reasons for the improvements seen in oral health:
- Introduction and widespread availability of fluoride toothpaste.
- Changed public and professional attitudes to tooth loss.
- Increased access to dental care.
- Development of dental technology, especially in relation to endodontics, crown and bridge techniques and latterly implants.

Implications of changes in oral health

The changes described have implications for both clinicians and commissioners of oral care.

Implications for clinicians

- Younger patients with essentially healthy dentitions may increasingly demand cosmetic and aesthetic treatments.
- Toothwear will increase and dentists will face the need to manage an increasing number of patients with worn dentitions (Figure 8.1).
- Increased tooth retention in association with gingival recession heightens the likelihood of root caries development.
- With age, the degree of periodontal attachment loss increases (Figure 6.4), so the proportion of older people with periodontal problems will increase.
- Most old people will in future have teeth, and in the majority of cases a good number of teeth. The number of old people in the population is increasing as the baby boomers born in the period 1946–64 become the aged population. People are living longer, so there will be more old people to treat, and nearly all of them will have teeth.
- If patients do eventually lose all of their teeth at an older age, adaptation to dentures can be a problem due to reduced muscle balance.
- Older people are likely to have co-morbidities that either affect their oral health or complicate the provision of oral care.
- In the past, performing simple extractions or construction of dentures in a domiciliary setting was relatively easy. It is more challenging to treat an older person who may have lost mental capacity due to dementia and who has toothache associated with a heavily restored dentition.

Implications for commissioners

- Oral health promotion needs for older dentate adults have to be considered, e.g. addressing changing diet on retirement.
- Skill-mix issues:
  - Use of hygienists and therapists to treat low-need younger people.
  - Target dentists' skills at more high-need older people.
- Training needs of future dental professionals may change, e.g. less frequent construction of complete dentures.
- The requirement to commission access to care for people in nursing and residential care homes.

10 International oral health

Figure 10.1 Average DMFT 12 year olds-European countries (2000-most recently available data).
Source: *WHO 2014. Reproduced with permission from the World Health Organization.*

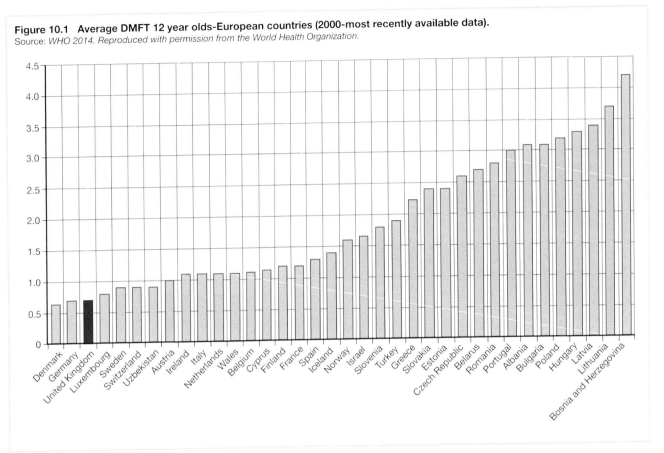

The World Health Organization and oral health

Previous chapters have looked at oral health in the United Kingdom. However, it is important to have an understanding of the epidemiology of oral disease across the world. The body responsible for securing an oversight of global oral health status is the World Health Organization (WHO). At intervals the WHO provides reports and commentaries on the state of oral health via the WHO Global Oral Health Programme. This is one of the technical programmes of its Department of Chronic Disease and Health Promotion.

A key issue in promoting oral health and securing access to dental care is resource allocation. In developing countries getting oral health onto the agenda can be a problem when there are other health issues that may be seen as more pressing. Recognition of the common risk factor approach (Chapter 21) to improving oral health allows oral disease prevention to be incorporated into wider health-promotion activities.

Global dental epidemiological data

Some countries, like the United Kingdom, have comprehensive arrangements for the collection of oral health data. In the United States, the National Health and Examination Survey (NHANES) is a programme of studies designed to assess the health and nutritional status of adults and children. The programme has been running since the early 1960s and at intervals includes the collection of data on the oral health of Americans. However, in many other countries oral health surveys are not conducted at regular intervals. In an attempt to standardize data-collection methods across the world, the WHO has issued guidance on the basic methods to be used in dental surveys. A copy is available to download from the WHO website (http://www.who.int/oral_health/publications/9789241548649/en/). A centre affiliated to the WHO at the University of Malmo in Sweden maintains a database on the oral health of countries across the world.

Oral disease – international perspective

Across the world dental caries and periodontal disease are the major contributors to oral ill health.

Dental caries

The WHO oral health database has been used to construct Figure 10.1. This shows the DMFT at age 12 in selected European countries, and demonstrates that relative to most of Europe, oral health at this age in the United Kingdom is very good. However, the wide variation seen across Europe is apparent from this graph. Oral health in Eastern European countries is worse by a factor of three than in the countries with the best oral health, which include the United Kingdom. This has implications for UK dentists, as children from Eastern Europe may migrate with their parents to the United Kingdom, leading dentists to see levels of decay in immigrant children that were last observed two and more decades ago.

In developing countries such as in much of Africa, historically levels of dental caries were low, due mainly to the low level of sugar present in traditional diets. However, as multinational food companies spread their operations across the world, cariogenic foods are increasingly within reach of all peoples in even the poorest of countries. Lack of exposure to fluoride in many countries coupled with increased exposure to sugar has seen high levels of tooth decay across the globe. In many Latin American countries, the mean DMFT at age 35–44 is over 14.

Periodontal disease

Severe periodontal disease, defined as a Community Periodontal Index Treatment Need (CPITN) score of 4 (i.e. pocket depth > 5.5 mm), affects 11.2% of the population worldwide – about 743 million people. The prevalence of severe periodontitis is remarkably similar around the world and is shown in Table 10.1.

Oral cancer

The prevalence of oral cancer varies markedly around the world and overall is the eighth most common cancer. In the United States the prevalence is estimated at 2.5 cases per 100,000 inhabitants. The highest rates of oral cancer are seen in south central Asia, where oral cancer is among the three most common types of cancer. This is largely attributed to the widespread habit of using betel and other smokeless tobacco products.

Noma (cancrum oris)

Noma is a disfiguring gangrenous condition that is seen most commonly in sub-Saharan Africa. The prevalence is estimated at 1 to 7 cases per 1000 population. It predominantly affects children and young people (2–16 years). The disease results in the destruction of the soft tissues of the face and the underlying bone. Risk factors are poverty, malnutrition, poor oral hygiene, residential proximity to livestock and infectious diseases such as measles and herpes viruses. It is thought that the resulting impaired immune system allows bacteria such as *Fusobacterium necrophorum* and *Prevotella intermedia* to destroy the facial tissues. Acute necrotizing gingivitis or ulcers arising from herpes virus infections may initiate the noma lesion. Untreated, 70–90% of patients will die.

HIV/AIDS and oral health

The WHO estimates that at the end of 2013 around 35 million people around the world were living with the human immunodeficiency virus (HIV). Infection with HIV predisposes the individual to oral infections due to weakened immune defence mechanisms. Common infections are candida (thrush), herpes simplex virus-1, herpes zoster, oral hairy leukoplakia and oral warts due to human papilloma virus, Kaposi's sarcoma, aphthous ulcers and xerostomia. Further facts on HIV are given in Table 10.2.

Advances in antiretroviral therapy mean that if they are diagnosed promptly, people infected with HIV can expect a near normal lifespan.

Table 10.1 Global prevalence of severe periodontitis (defined as CPITN = 4) in 2010

Location	Prevalence (%) of severe periodontitis – CPITN = 4, pocket depth > 5.5 mm (2010)
Global	11.2
Asia Pacific, high income	8.0
Asia	
Central	13.8
East	10.4
South	10.2
South East	13.1
Australasia	14.9
Caribbean	8.6
Europe	
Central	12.1
Eastern	14.0
Western	9.4
Latin America	
Andean	15.2
Central	15.1
Southern	20.4
Tropical	18.5
North Africa/Middle East	10.4
North America, high income	7.2
Oceania	4.2
Sub-Saharan Africa	
Central	13.3
East	20.1
Southern	9.2
West	9.3

Source: *Kassebaum 2014. Reproduced with permission from Sage Publications.*

Table 10.2 Facts about human immunodeficiency virus

HIV globally	
Number of people living with HIV/AIDS worldwide	
End of 2013	35 (33.2–37.2) million
End of 2001	29.8 (28.1–31.9) million
Of the global total in 2013, number of people living with HIV in sub-Saharan Africa	24.7 million – 71% of global total
Global number of people who died of an AIDS-related illness in 2013	1.5 million

HIV in the UK	
Number of people living with HIV/AIDS in the UK	
End of 2012	98,000
Diagnosed and accessing care	77,610
Undiagnosed	21,900
Prevalence of HIV in the UK (2012)	1.5 per 1000 population
Men who have sex with men (MSM)	47 per 1000 MSM
Heterosexual men and women (Black African men and women are at increased risk)	38 per 1000 in this group
Injecting drug users	13 per 1000 users
Pregnant women	2.2 per 1000 pregnant women
UK-born pregnant women	0.5 per 1000 pregnant women
Sub-Saharan Africa born pregnant women	23 per 1000 pregnant women

Sources: *Data from Public Health England 2013 and from WHO 2015.*

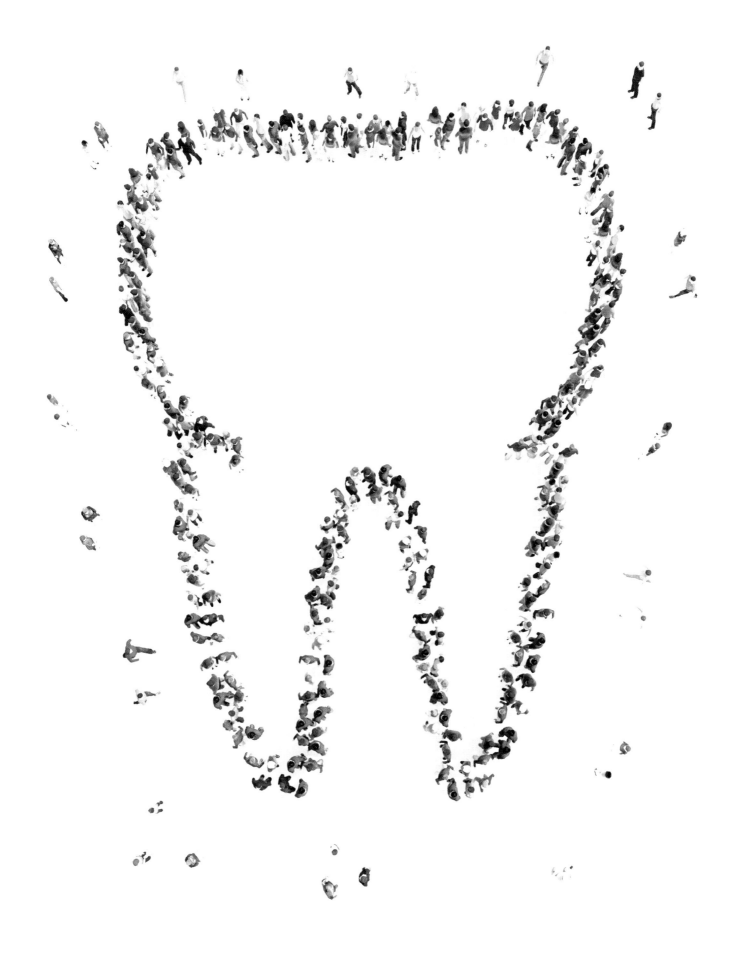

Evidence-based dentistry

Chapters

11 Study design

Figure 11.1 Study design in the research process

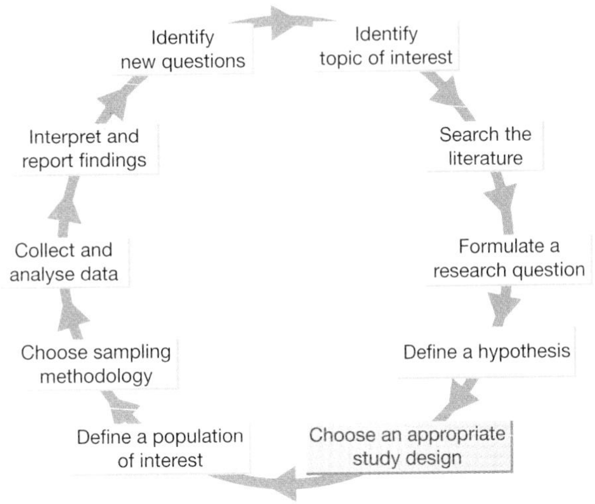

Identify new questions → Identify topic of interest → Search the literature → Formulate a research question → Define a hypothesis → Choose an appropriate study design → Define a population of interest → Choose sampling methodology → Collect and analyse data → Interpret and report findings → (Identify new questions)

Figure 11.2 Observational/interventional studies

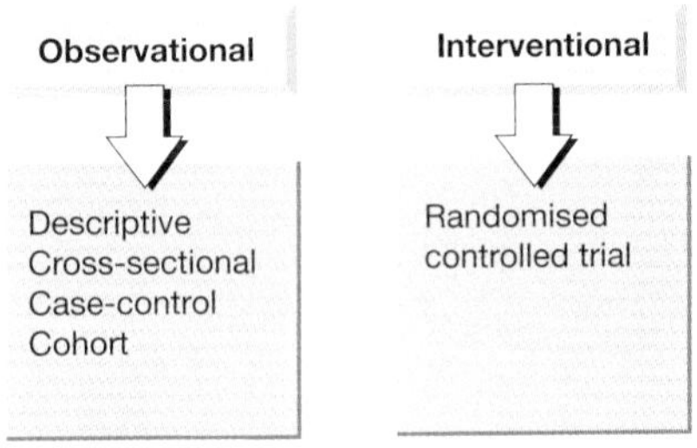

Observational
Descriptive
Cross-sectional
Case-control
Cohort

Interventional
Randomised controlled trial

Figure 11.3 Time and study design

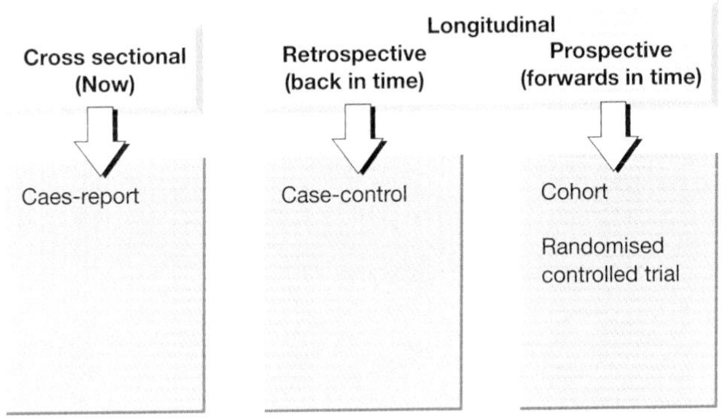

Cross sectional (Now)
Caes-report

Longitudinal

Retrospective (back in time)
Case-control

Prospective (forwards in time)
Cohort

Randomised controlled trial

Figure 11.4 Primary and secondary studies

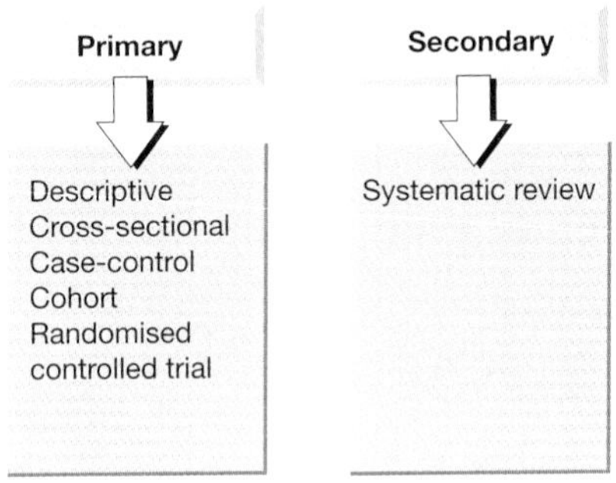

Primary
Descriptive
Cross-sectional
Case-control
Cohort
Randomised controlled trial

Secondary
Systematic review

Dental Public Health at a Glance, First Edition. Ivor G. Chestnutt.
© 2016 John Wiley & Sons, Ltd. Published 2016 by John Wiley & Sons, Ltd.

Study design

Study design requires an understanding of the different approaches that may be taken to answer a research question. How study design fits into the research process is shown in Figure 11.1. Different research questions require different types of study design. The most significant difference between different types of study is the degree to which they control for outside factors such as **bias** and **confounding**. A good understanding of study design is fundamental to good research and critical appraisal skills. The principal types of study design are shown in Table 11.1.

Observational and interventional studies

Studies can be described as **observational** or **interventional** (Figure 11.2). In observational studies no attempt is made to alter or interfere with the participants or the environment – as the name suggests, the study is confined to recording facts purely by observation. In interventional studies, the researchers manipulate the participants or their environment in some way – they conduct an experiment.

Time and study design

The time period over which a study is conducted is another fundamental issue in study design. Studies can be described as **cross-sectional**, so carried out at a point in time. **Longitudinal** studies follow participants over time, either by looking backward from the present time (**retrospective**) or looking forward (**prospective**) (Figure 11.3). The issue of time is crucial, as cause and effect can only be inferred from longitudinal studies.

Primary and secondary research

Studies can be further categorized as **primary** or **secondary** research (Figure 11.4). In primary research, new data are gathered from or about participants or their environment. Secondary research involves the generation of new data from existing studies. The generation of evidence by combining results from different studies (as occurs in a systematic review) is secondary research.

Cause, effect and association

It is crucial to remember that just because two factors are shown to be associated in a study, it does not mean that one necessarily causes the other or vice versa. The following factors, described by Bradford-Hill, can be used to infer that a relationship is causal. As an example, the relationship between cigarette smoking and periodontal attachment loss is used in this way.

Table 11.1 Types of study design

Type of study	
Case report (descriptive) Cross-sectional Case-control Cohort Randomized controlled trial Systematic review	More robust study design More controlled for bias and confounding factors

Strength of the association

A causal relationship can be inferred if the condition of interest occurs much more frequently in people exposed to the risk factor. This holds true in the case of cigarette smoking and periodontal attachment loss. Periodontal pockets are more common in people who smoke tobacco.

Dose-response

A relationship is more likely to be causal if the extent of the disease is linked to the degree of exposure to the causative factor. Periodontal attachment loss is worse in heavy smokers than light smokers, who in turn have more attachment loss than non-smokers.

Change in risk factor

Removal of the suspected causative factor should lead to a reduction in the disease, or at least no further progression. Former smokers have less periodontal disease than those who continue to smoke.

Temporal relationship

A causal relationship is more likely if the disease in question occurs after exposure to the suspected risk factor. This is difficult to demonstrate using the example of periodontal disease and tobacco smoking, but could be shown in a cohort study.

Consistency

A causal relationship is more likely if the relationship between the disease and suspected causative factor has been shown to hold true in multiple studies. So in the example of periodontal disease and smoking, studies conducted in different sites around the world have demonstrated that periodontal disease is worse in smokers.

Specificity

In a causal relationship, a postulated causal factor should lead to the disease in question and no other. Clearly, this is not the case in the example of cigarette smoking, which is causally related to many diseases and conditions other than periodontal disease.

Biological plausibility

If a biological mechanism can be proposed for the suspected causal factor, that strengthens the likelihood of a causal relationship. It has been shown that nicotine has vasoconstrictive effects on gingival blood vessels and has detrimental effects on neutrophils. These have been postulated as mechanisms whereby smoking interferes with the host defence mechanisms, thereby predisposing to periodontal attachment loss.

Experiment

It is possible to demonstrate a causal relationship by experiment – that is the basis of a randomized controlled trial (Chapters 15 and 16). However, this can only be done where the action is to prevent disease or to remove a suspected causative factor. In the smoking and periodontal disease example, it would be possible (although practically difficult) to conduct an experiment to examine the effects of stopping smoking on periodontal health. It would of course be unethical to look at the relationship in reverse; that is, to encourage people to smoke in order to examine the effects of smoking tobacco on the periodontal tissues.

12 Case reports and cross-sectional studies

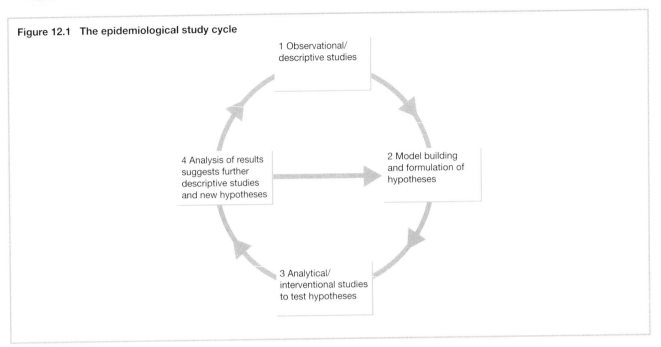

Figure 12.1 The epidemiological study cycle

1 Observational/ descriptive studies

2 Model building and formulation of hypotheses

3 Analytical/ interventional studies to test hypotheses

4 Analysis of results suggests further descriptive studies and new hypotheses

Case reports

The simplest type of research report, a **case report**, is a description of a single case or series of cases, typically of an unusual finding or alternative means of managing a condition. It is often accompanied by a brief literature review that describes similar cases reported previously and a discussion of the implications of the case or cases reported.

Advantages of case reports

• Useful for describing unusual events or rarely encountered situations.
• Educational – may help those who subsequently encounter a similar case.

• May be the first report of a never before recognized condition – for example hairy leukoplakia, one of the oral manifestations of Acquired Immune Deficiency Syndrome (AIDS), was initially reported in a series of case reports.

Disadvantages of case reports

• They are reports of only one or a few cases and are anecdotal and subjective in nature.
• There is no control for bias and confounding.
• They cannot be used to draw conclusions about the cause, prevention or definitive management of the condition described.

Dental Public Health at a Glance, First Edition. Ivor G. Chestnutt.
© 2016 John Wiley & Sons, Ltd. Published 2016 by John Wiley & Sons, Ltd.

Cross-sectional studies (surveys)

Cross-sectional studies or surveys are commonly used in dental public health. They can be used to:

- Estimate the prevalence of a disease/condition/habit.
- Report the current health status of a defined group.
- Establish reference ranges.
- Determine the cut-off points for a diagnostic test.

The most common form of cross-sectional survey is the series of epidemiological surveys that are carried out to determine the oral health status of a representative sample of the population.

In the United Kingdom there are two major series of surveys.

Decennial surveys of child and adult oral health

These surveys are commissioned by the Departments of Health in the United Kingdom.

The child surveys have been conducted in 1973, 1983, 1993, 2003 and 2013.

The adult surveys have been conducted in 1968 (England and Wales only), 1978, 1988, 1998 and 2009.

British Association for the Study of Community Dentistry surveys

Since 1986, a series of surveys, focusing mainly on children but more recently also including limited surveys of specific adult groups, have been undertaken by the Community/Salaried Dental Services. These studies are commissioned by local health bodies (Health Boards in Scotland and Wales, Local Authorities in England). The criteria for these surveys have been drawn up by the British Association for the Study of Community Dentistry and are designed to guide the sampling procedure and criteria used to record the clinical conditions being measured – primarily dental caries.

International oral health surveys

In the United States, the National Health and Nutrition Examination Survey (NHANES) comprises a series of interviews and physical examinations of a representative sample of the US population. This includes oral health. The programme has been running since the 1960s.

The World Health Organization maintains a database of international oral health surveys.

In addition to these series of cross sectional surveys, one-off surveys, which can take the form of clinical examinations or questionnaires – either administered in person, by telephone, by post or online – can be used to gather data at a given point in time.

Advantages of cross-sectional studies (surveys)

- Can be used to determine how common a condition is – the prevalence (Chapter 3).
- Can be used to determine access to services at a given point in time.
- Can be used to gather current opinion (opinion poll).
- Are easy to conduct compared to longitudinal studies.

Disadvantages of cross-sectional studies (surveys)

- As they lack a temporal element, cross-sectional studies cannot be used to make causal inferences.

Trend data

From a series of cross-sectional surveys it is possible to determine trends. As an example, from the Adult Dental Health Surveys it has been possible to show that the proportion of the population who are edentulous (have lost all of their teeth) has decreased from 30% in 1978 to 6% in 2009. It should be noted that although trends can be established from a series of cross-sectional studies, this does not equate to disease increment, as different individuals are involved in successive surveys.

Ecological studies

Ecological studies are a form of cross-sectional study, where populations or whole communities form the unit of analysis. In ecological studies, cause and effect are often determined by comparing geographical areas. Many useful observations have been made from ecological studies, but they are prone to confounding caused by differences in the age and gender structure of the populations being compared. For this reason the use of **standardized data** is important (Chapter 3). In dental public health, investigations of the effects of water fluoridation are often in the form of ecological studies.

An important issue is the **ecological fallacy**. This occurs when conclusions are drawn from groups of individuals and applied to individuals. As an example, suppose data are available detailing the prevalence of dental caries in a series of school classes in a town. If we were to visit the class with the highest caries score and select a child from that class and say that he/she had a high caries score, that would be an example of an ecological fallacy. Because the caries level in the class as a whole is high, it does not follow that an individual child picked at random from that class will have a high caries experience. That child could well be one of the few with a low caries score.

The epidemiological study cycle

The epidemiological study cycle demonstrates how observational studies can be used to inform theory and models that can subsequently be investigated using interventional studies (Figure 12.1).

A good example of the epidemiological study cycle are the studies conducted in the United States in the first half of the twentieth century on water fluoridation (Chapter 26). Observational studies of dental fluorosis, the association between the level of fluoride in the water supply and caries prevalence led to the hypothesis that by adding fluoride to the public water supply, the prevalence of dental caries could be reduced. This theory was tested using an intervention study and water fluoridation was shown to be an effective means of preventing dental caries (detail in Table 26.1).

13 Case-control studies

Figure 13.1 Case-control and cohort studies

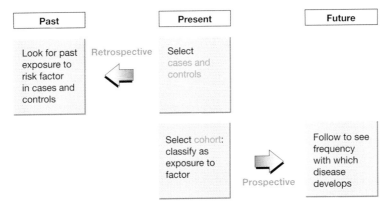

Past	Present	Future
Look for past exposure to risk factor in cases and controls	← Retrospective Select cases and controls	
	Select cohort: classify as exposure to factor	Prospective → Follow to see frequency with which disease develops

Figure 13.2 Case-control study

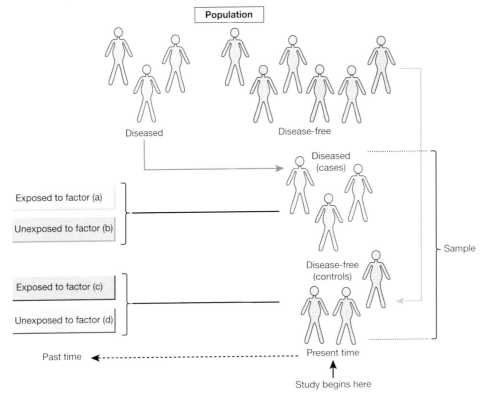

Population

Diseased   Disease-free

Diseased (cases)

Exposed to factor (a)
Unexposed to factor (b)

Disease-free (controls)

Exposed to factor (c)
Unexposed to factor (d)

Sample

Past time ←------------------- Present time

Study begins here

Figure 13.3 Analysis of a case-control study

Reported as an odds ratio

$$\text{Odds ratio} = \frac{\text{Odds of being a case in exposed group}}{\text{Odds of being a case in unexposed group}}$$

	Exposed to factor		
	Yes	No	Total
Disease status			
Case	a	b	a+b
Control	c	d	c+d
Total	a+c	b+d	a+b+c+d

$$\text{Odds}_{exp} = \frac{\left[\dfrac{a}{a+c}\right]}{\left[\dfrac{c}{a+c}\right]} = \frac{a}{c}$$

$$\text{Odds}_{unexp} = \frac{\left[\dfrac{b}{b+d}\right]}{\left[\dfrac{d}{b+d}\right]} = \frac{b}{d}$$

Therefore estimated odds ratio =

$$\frac{a/c}{b/d} = \frac{a \times d}{b \times c}$$

Typically reported as odds ratio and confidence interval of the odds ratio

Dental Public Health at a Glance, First Edition. Ivor G. Chestnutt.
© 2016 John Wiley & Sons, Ltd. Published 2016 by John Wiley & Sons, Ltd.

Case-control studies

A case-control study is an observational study design that at the outset selects **cases** (individuals with the disease or condition of interest) and matches these with **controls** (individuals who do not have the disease or condition of interest). Cases and controls are usually matched for possible confounding factors such as age and gender. This means that the case and control groups will have approximately the same age and gender and so the influence of these parameters is reduced. The researchers then examine the difference in exposure to suspected risk/aetiological factors of both cases and controls. Case-control studies are **retrospective** in nature (Figure 13.1). They focus on events that have happened at or prior to selection of the participants.

Analysis of a case-control study

A 2 × 2 table can be constructed from which the odds of being a case in the exposed group can be compared with the odds of being a case in the unexposed group. From this an **estimated odds ratio** can be calculated (Figures 13.2 and 13.3). Odds ratios are usually presented ± the 95% confidence interval (CI). This represents the degree of certainty surrounding the estimated odds ratio. An odds ratio of 1 means that there is no difference in risk between the case and control groups. If the odds ratio is greater than 1 then exposure to the suspected risk factor implies a greater risk of developing the disease/condition being investigated. An odds ratio of less than 1 implies that exposure to the factor under investigation actually reduces risk of the disease/condition.

Advantages of case-control studies

- Generally relatively quick, cheap and easy to perform.
- More than one risk factor can be investigated.
- Can be conducted with relatively few cases.
- Good for investigating the cause of rare diseases (because possible to identify all cases from more than one site).
- No loss to follow-up.

Disadvantages of case-control studies

- Require availability of historical record of exposures. If this has not been recorded or there is bias in recording it can lead to incorrect assumptions about exposure to the suspected risk factor.

Box 13.1 Example of a case-control study

Occupational exposures and risk of oesophageal cancer by histological type: A case-control study in eastern Spain.
Santibañez, M. et al. (2008) Occupational and Environmental Medicine, 65:774–81.

OBJECTIVE: To explore the relationship between occupations and specific occupational exposures and oesophageal cancer (OC) by histological type.

A multicentre hospital-based case-control study was conducted in two Mediterranean provinces of Spain. Occupational, socio-demographic and lifestyle information was collected from 185 newly diagnosed male oesophageal cancer patients (147 squamous cell, 38 adenocarcinoma) and 285 frequency matched controls.

RESULTS: For the squamous cell variety, statistically significant associations were found for waiters and bartenders (OR 8.18, 95% CI 1.98–33.75) and miners, shotfirers, stone cutters and carvers (OR 10.78, 95% CI 1.24–93.7) in relation to other occupations. For the adenocarcinoma variety, statistically significant associations were observed for carpenters and joiners (OR 9.69), animal producers and related workers (OR 5.61) and building workers and related electricians (OR 8.26), although these observations were based on a low number of cases.

Source: Santibañez et al. 2008. Reproduced with permission from BMJ Publishing Group.

- **Recall bias**, which occurs when cases have an erroneous memory of exposure to risk factors. They may for example put greater emphasis on exposure to a suspected risk factor than do controls, thereby biasing the exposure record.
- An adequate control group may be difficult to define or obtain.

The example in Box 13.1 demonstrates the use of a case-control study to determine the impact of occupational exposures on cancer of the oesophagus. It can be seen that waiters and bartenders are 8.18 times more likely to develop squamous cell carcinoma of the oesophagus. Presumably this may be through occupational exposure to tobacco smoke or perhaps access to alcohol or a combination of both. However, the 95% confidence interval is wide and ranges from 1.98 to 33.75, meaning that the risk of waiters and bartenders developing oesophageal cancer could be from twice that of non-waiters and bartenders to nearly 34 times. The confidence intervals are wide because of the small number of cases. A greater number of cases in the study would provide a more precise estimate of the odds ratio and the 95% confidence intervals would be narrower.

14 Cohort studies

Figure 14.1 Cohort study

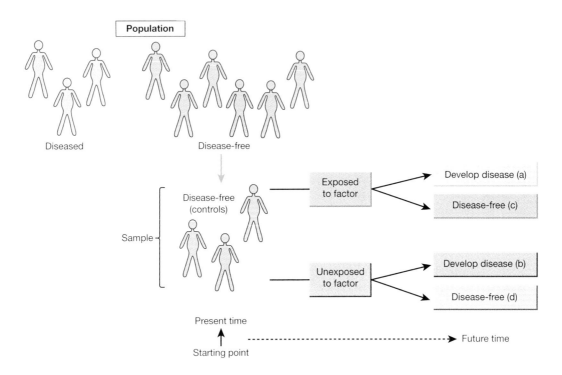

Figure 14.2 Analysis of a cohort study

Because patients are followed can determine risk (compare: estimated odds in case/control studies)

Estimated risk of disease in the exposed group

$$risk_{exp} = a/(a+c)$$

Estimated risk of disease in the unexposed group

$$risk_{unexp} = b/(b+d)$$

Estimated relative risk

$$= risk_{exp}/risk_{unexp}$$

$$= \frac{a/(a+c)}{b/(b+d)}$$

Results are expressed as relative risk plus confidence intervals

	Exposed to factor		
	Yes	No	Total
Disease status			
Yes	a	b	a+b
No	c	d	c+d
Total	a+c	b+d	a+b+c+d

Dental Public Health at a Glance, First Edition. Ivor G. Chestnutt.
© 2016 John Wiley & Sons, Ltd. Published 2016 by John Wiley & Sons, Ltd.

Cohort studies

A **cohort study** is a form of observational study in which the participants are followed over a period of time from the starting point. A cohort study is **prospective** in nature. That is, participants are followed over time (Figures 13.1 and 14.1). At the beginning of the study the participants are free of the disease/condition of interest, but vary in their exposure to possible risk factors. Over time, they are examined and separated into those who do and those who do not develop the condition of interest. The differences in exposure to risk factors are observed and the **relative risk** of developing the disease depending on exposure to the examined risk factors can be calculated.

Analysis of a cohort study

A 2 × 2 table can be constructed from which it is possible to calculate the estimated risk of developing the disease in those exposed to the risk factor. The estimated risk of developing the disease in those unexposed to the risk factor can also be calculated. The relative risk can therefore be calculated as the risk in the exposed group divided by the risk in the unexposed group (Figure 14.2). This is usually presented along with the 95% confidence intervals, which give an estimate of the degree of precision of the estimated relative risk.

Advantages of cohort studies

• The time sequence of exposure to the suspected risk factor and development of the disease can be determined.
• More than one outcome can be considered.
• This design allows the risk of disease to be measured directly.
• It is possible, given sufficient resources, to measure information about exposure to risk factors in detail and also to examine exposure to a range of risk factors.
• There is likely to be less chance of **recall** and **selection bias** than in case-control studies.
• Exposure is measured prior to outcome and so helps avoid bias.

Disadvantages of cohort studies

• Because the participants have to be followed up for a long period of time, cohort studies are expensive to conduct.
• If the disease or condition is rare, it is necessary to follow up a large number of individuals (hence case-control studies are generally better for investigating rare conditions).

BOX 14.1 Example of a cohort study

Cannabis smoking and periodontal disease among young adults
Thomson, W.M. et al. (2008) *Journal of the American Medical Association*, 229:525–32.
   OBJECTIVE: To examine the effect of cannabis use on periodontal attachment loss.
   METHODS: Prospective cohort study of the general population, with cannabis use determined at ages 18, 21, 26 and 32 years and dental examinations conducted at ages 26 and 32 years.
   RESULTS: After controlling for tobacco smoking (measured in pack-years), gender, irregular use of dental services and dental plaque, the relative risk estimates for the highest cannabis exposure group were as follows: 1.6 (95% confidence interval [CI], 1.2–2.2) for having 1 or more sites with 4 mm or greater clinical attachment loss; 3.1 (95% CI, 1.5–6.4) for having 1 or more sites with 5 mm or greater clinical attachment loss; and 2.2 (95% CI, 1.2–3.9) for having incident attachment loss (in comparison with those who had never smoked cannabis).

Source: Thomson et al. 2008. Reproduced with permission from American Medical Association.

• Loss of participants over time can introduce bias. This is particularly a problem if the loss is linked to a risk factor.
• It is important to maintain consistency of measuring either exposure to the risk factor or the disease of interest for the duration of the study (which may in some cases be years).
• Disease outcome or risk factors may themselves change over time.

An example of a Cohort study is shown in Box 14.1.

This study involved a cohort of just over 1000 individuals born in Dunedin, New Zealand in 1972/73 and who have been followed since birth. In this report the effect of reported cannabis use on periodontal attachment loss was examined. Tobacco smoking, gender, irregular use of dental services and dental plaque are known to be risk factors for periodontal attachment loss. These factors are 'controlled for' using advanced statistical techniques such as multivariate analysis. This allows the contribution of cannabis to attachment loss to be estimated taking into account the other known risk factors. The authors have concluded that for the heaviest users of cannabis, the risk of having 1 or more sites with 4 mm or greater clinical attachment loss was 1.6. This means that heavy cannabis users are 1.6 times more likely to experience this degree of attachment loss. The 95% confidence interval ranges from 1.2 to 2.2, meaning that while the risk overall was estimated at 1.6, it could be as low as 1.2 or as high as 2.2. In fact it is 95% certain that the increased risk lies between these values. Because the 95% CI does not include 1, it can be concluded that the risk observed is statistically significant.

15 Randomized controlled trials

Figure 15.1 Randomized control trial

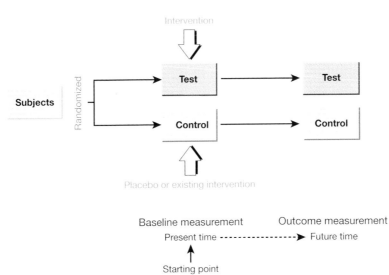

Figure 15.2 Consort Diagram - to show participant flow through a trial. Source: *Schulz et al. 2010. Reproduced with permission from BMJ Publishing Group.*

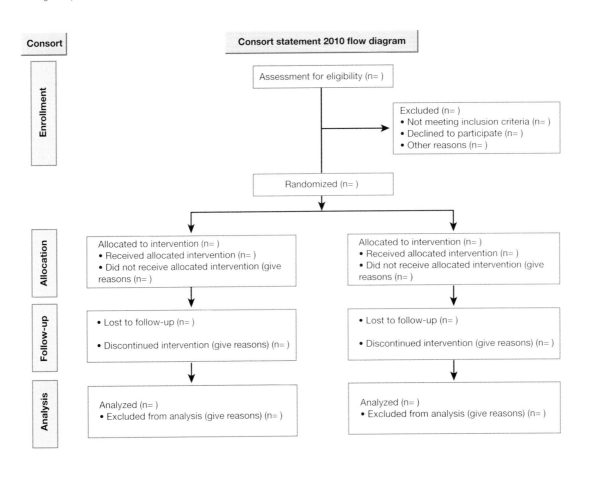

Dental Public Health at a Glance, First Edition. Ivor G. Chestnutt.
© 2016 John Wiley & Sons, Ltd. Published 2016 by John Wiley & Sons, Ltd.

A randomized controlled trial (RCT) is an **interventional study** and is **prospective** in nature (Figure 15.1). Study participants are identified according to predefined inclusion criteria. The participants are then assigned at **random** to either a **test group** or a **control group**. The test group then receives the intervention under test, while the control group receives no intervention, a **placebo** intervention or an existing treatment. The participants are followed for a period of time and the **outcome** measured at the end. The change from baseline in both test and control groups is measured. The test and control groups are then compared to determine whether there is any **difference in outcome** in the test and control groups. In this way a conclusion can be reached on whether the intervention or treatment applied to the test group had a more desirable outcome than the intervention received by the control group.

Analysis of a randomized controlled trial

The type of analysis undertaken in a randomized controlled trial will depend on the nature of the outcome measure used. The general principle is the application of a statistical test to determine whether the difference in outcome observed between the test and control group at the end of the study is likely to have occurred by chance or is likely to be a true difference.

It is then necessary to determine whether the difference is of **clinical significance**. It is possible for the difference to be statistically significant – that is, for it to be true and not simply have occurred by chance. However, it is possible that the difference is small and not likely to be of greater clinical benefit over the intervention received by the control group.

Advantages of randomized controlled trials

• Are considered the **'gold standard'** of study design, largely because of the degree to which they can control for bias and confounding factors.
• Allow randomization and can therefore minimize the effect of confounding.
• Can be 'blind' and therefore minimize the effect of bias.
• Are often multicentre – that is, participants are recruited from more than one site.
• Participants in RCTs get excellent care (even if in the control group).

Disadvantages of randomized controlled trials

• Expensive to conduct.
• Require specialist skills to organize and conduct.
• Recruitment of sufficient numbers of study participants in a defined period of time can be a challenge.
• Participants can be lost to follow-up.
• RCTs can only be used to examine interventions with a positive outcome for the participants. It is unethical to use an RCT design to examine the aetiology of disease. So for example, while it is appropriate to test the anti-caries effect of fluoride-containing toothpaste in an RCT, it would be unethical to demonstrate the cariogenic effect of sugar using an RCT design.

Issues relating to randomized controlled trials

Randomization

The term 'random' in RCT relates to the manner in which participants are allocated to either the test or control group. Each participant should have an equal chance of being allocated or **randomized** to either the test or control group.

Usually participants are randomized on an individual basis. However, sometimes participants are randomized in groups or '**clusters**', for example, schools or classrooms within a school. **Cluster randomized controlled trials** will require more participants and the clustering effect needs to be accounted for in the analysis of the trial outcome.

Stratification

While individuals are allocated to a trial arm at random, it is important that before the trial begins, the test and control groups are as alike as possible. For example, in a clinical trial of a fluoride-containing toothpaste, the test and control groups should not differ significantly in terms of caries prevalence, number of males and females or age of participants. This is achieved by a process called **stratification**. In critically appraising a clinical trial, it is important to look for a table that at **baseline** compares important possible confounding factors between test and control groups.

Blinding

Blinding (or allocation concealment) is the process whereby the study group to which a participant is allocated is hidden from the participant, the experimenter conducting the outcome measurement or both. When only the participant is unaware of the intervention they are receiving this is known as '**single blind**'. When both participant and experimenter are unaware, this is known as '**double blind**'. In a '**triple-blind**' study the statistician carrying out the study analysis is also unaware which of the groups is receiving the test intervention and which is receiving the control intervention.

Trial arm

The term 'arm' is used to describe a group receiving the same intervention. In a classical clinical trial there are two arms, the test group and the control group (Figure 15.1). However, some trials can have more than two arms – as many as six in some studies, although these require very large numbers of participants.

Training and calibration

It is important that the experimenters measuring the study outcome do so in a reproducible and consistent manner. To achieve this, the clinicians recording the study outcome undergo training in the use of the instrument or index (Chapter 4) employed to measure the outcome. To ensure that they are scoring the outcome in a similar fashion, a **calibration exercise** is carried out where the examiners all measure the same patient or photograph of an outcome measure. The level of agreement among the examiners can be determined statistically and is reported as a **Kappa score**. A score of 1 indicates perfect agreement (this seldom occurs) and a score of 0 represents no agreement. Calibration of examiners is particularly important when study participants are recruited at multiple sites. For example, the FiCTION clinical trial (Innes et al., 2013), which is examining the clinical and cost effectiveness of restoring primary teeth compared with no treatment, is recruiting children across Britain.

It is important that all of the examiners assess the outcomes in a consistent fashion. The CONSORT standard for reporting RCTs is outlined in Figure 15.2.

Randomized controlled trials II: Split mouth and cross-over studies

Figure 16.1 Diagrammatic representation of a split-mouth randomized controlled trial

Restorative material A placed on right hand side in 50% of study participants and on left hand side in 50% (vice-versa with material B). Both materials are therefore tested in the same oral environment

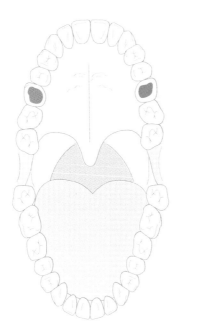
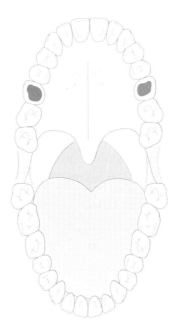

Figure 16.2 Diagrammatic representation of a cross-over study

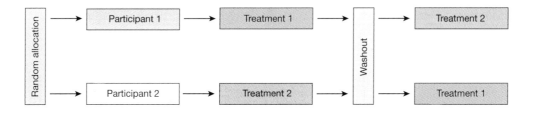

In addition to the conventional parallel, two-arm randomized controlled trial (Chapter 15, Figure 15.1), there are two other forms of interventional study design that are encountered in dental research. These are both forms of controlled clinical trials in which the participants act as both test and control: a split mouth trial and a cross-over trial.

Split mouth clinical trial

In a study of this design, a participant receives two interventions simultaneously, the test on one side of the mouth and the control on the contralateral (same arch, opposite side) or ipsilateral (opposite arch, same side) side (Figure 16.1). The side that receives the test treatment is decided at random, but overall 50% of participants will have the test intervention on the right side and 50% on the left. This minimizes any effect of bias due to the treatment being on the left- or right-hand side. Occasionally the control site may be ipsilateral (i.e. test sites are in mandible and maxilla on same side of the mouth). Some studies have tested four interventions, one in each quadrant of the mouth. Split mouth studies are most useful for investigating restorative dental materials. It is important that 'cross-over' effects are considered before utilizing a split mouth design. For example, it would not be appropriate to test a fluoride-releasing glass-ionomer restorative material in a split mouth study. Fluoride leach may affect the control site on the contra- or ipsilateral side.

Advantages of a split mouth trial

• Test and control interventions tested in the same intraoral environment, thereby helping to control confounding factors.
• Fewer participants needed.

Disadvantages of a split mouth trial

• Statistical analysis needs to account for the fact that the sites are clustered/nested within one individual and are therefore not independent, and paired tests should be used.
• Need to recruit participants who require the intervention in two contra- (or ipsilateral) sites.
An example of a split mouth study can be found in Box 16.1.

This study investigated the effect of bevelling cavity preparations in primary teeth using a split mouth design.

Cross-over trial

In a study of this design, the participant receives both test and control treatment, but in series; that is, one after the other. An example would be a study on the anti-calculus properties of a toothpaste (Figure 16.2). Following a scale and polish, the study participant uses the test toothpaste for a period (in this example about three months) and the amount of new calculus that has developed is measured. The participant then uses a standard toothpaste for a period (in this example one month) to allow any 'hangover' effects of the test product to dissipate. Following a further scale and polish, the participant then uses the control toothpaste for a similar period to that for which they used the test treatment. The amount of new calculus that has developed is measured and compared with the test product. One half of the study participants will receive the test toothpaste first, while the other half will have the control product first, to minimize any order effects.

Advantages of a cross-over trial

• Test and control interventions are tested in the same participants, so fewer participants are required.
• Patients act as their own control, so confounding factors are minimized.

Disadvantages of a cross-over trial

• Can only be used to test outcomes that are recurrent and reversible, e.g. accumulation of dental plaque and calculus.
• Results are nested within participants and so more complex statistical analysis is required.
• Because treatments are tested in series (i.e. one after the other) the study lasts longer than a parallel study design.
An example of a cross-over study can be found in Box 16.2. Box 16.3 describes analysis of randomized controlled trials.

Box 16.2 Example of a cross-over study

Fasting state and episodes of vomiting in children receiving nitrous oxide for dental treatment.
Kupietzky, A. et al. (2008) *Pediatric Dentistry*, 30:414–19
PURPOSE: The purpose of this controlled cross-over study was to determine the frequency of vomiting during nitrous oxide/oxygen analgesia (NOA) and assess the relationship between fasting status and vomiting.
METHODS: 113 children (64 male, 49 female), ranging in age from 24–160 months (mean = 74) and a mean weight of 23 kg (range 11–60 kg), participated in the study. At the initial examination, subjects were randomly assigned to be either fasting on the first appointment and non-fasting during the second appointment, or non-fasting for the first appointment and fasting for the second.
RESULTS: The average time interval between eating and treatment in the fasting sessions was 6 hours and in the non-fasting group 1 hour before treatment. Vomiting occurred in only one subject, immediately after cessation of treatment, resulting in a frequency of 1% of subjects or 0.5% of sessions. No other differences were found between fasting and non-fasting subjects.

Source: *Kupietzky et al. 2008.*

Box 16.1 Example of a split mouth study

Split mouth randomized controlled clinical trial of bevelled cavity preparations in primary molars: an 18-Month follow up.
Oliveria, C.A. et al. (2008) *Journal of Dentistry*, 36:754–8
METHODS: A total of 94 Class I cavity preparations were performed in the carious primary molars of 32 children aged 4–10 years. Two cavity designs were used: conventional conservative preparation (G1) and modified preparation with cavo-surface bevel (G2). All teeth were restored using a resin composite material.
RESULTS: Bevel cavity design preparations did not improve the success of composite restorations in primary molars over 18 months.

Source: *Oliveria et al. 2008. Reproduced with permission from Elsevier.*

Box 16.3 Analysis of randomized controlled trials

Per protocol analysis – At the conclusion of an RCT only those participants who adhered to the published protocol are included in the analysis.
Intention to treat analysis – At the conclusion of an RCT, the outcome data for all participants (when available) is analysed according to the group to which they were allocated, irrespective of whether or not they adhered strictly to the trial protocol. This is the preferred form of analysis as it is less likely to introduce bias and also more likely to be reflective of 'real world' results. The main difficulty is having available outcome data for participants who fail to complete the trial.

17 Systematic reviews and meta-analysis

Figure 17.1 Forest plot – used to present outcome of meta-analysis

Studies with mean to the left of no-effect line indicate intervention not effective

In this example 7 studies contributed to the meta-analysis. 5 suggested a positive effect, 2 studies suggested no effect. Overall the meta-analysis suggests a definite positive effect

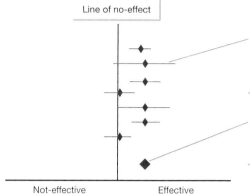

Line of no-effect

Each horizontal line represents a single study, the diamond is the mean odds ratio and the line represents the 95% Confidence Interval. Wide confidence intervals suggest a study with small number of participants

This large diamond represents the overall estimate effect. The centre of the diamond is mean effect, the width is the overall 95% Confidence Interval

Not-effective   Effective

Figure 17.2 PRISMA flow diagram. Source: *Moher et al. 2009. Reproduced under the terms of the Creative Commons Attribution Licence CC-BY.*

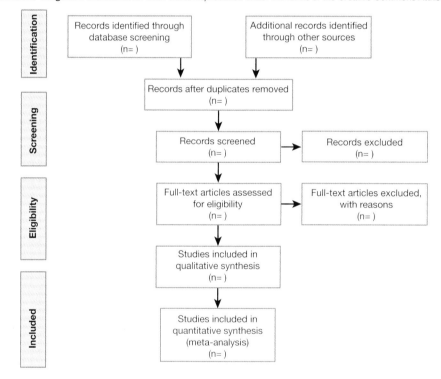

Figure 17.3 Funnel plot: (a) no publication bias, (b) publication bias

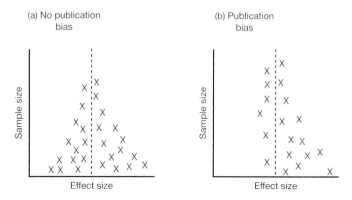

Publication bias – occurs when only a part of the existing data are available.
Publication can occur because journals are more likely to publish positive results and researchers may not seek publication of negative results.
The presence of publication bias can be detected using a funnel plot.
A funnel plot which is symmetrical about the mean and looks like an upside down funnel suggests no publication bias (a).
When the bottom left portion of the plot is missing– publication bias should be suspected (b).
The detection of publication bias is useful in interpreting the evidence but difficult to correct for.

Systematic review

A systematic review is a form of secondary research in which existing information is searched for in a highly organized fashion according to a predefined protocol. Efforts are made to identify not only information published in standard academic journals, but also that from the 'grey literature', not controlled by commercial publishers. Data are extracted from individual studies. Provided that a common outcome measure has been used and that there are sufficient studies, data can be combined statistically (meta-analysis) to give an overall effect. The typical steps in conducting a systematic review are shown in Table 17.1.

Advantages of systematic reviews

• Provide an overall summary of the effectiveness of an intervention or contribution of a risk factor to a disease/condition.

• Include the 'grey literature', unpublished studies.
• Include studies published in languages other than English.
• Overcome bias inherent in traditional narrative reviews, where the search strategy, inclusion and exclusion criteria and method for reaching a conclusion are not transparent.
• Development and use have been greatly encouraged by the Cochrane Collaboration (Chapter 18).

Limitations of systematic reviews

• Are reliant on a sufficient number of studies having been conducted with a similar outcome measure.
• The proper conduct of a systematic review requires researchers with a range of skills, e.g. literature search skills, as well as statisticians, research methodologists and clinicians.

Table 17.1 Steps in conducting a systematic review

Stage	Process
Identify topic for review and agree a clearly defined research question(s)	It is important to identify a clearly defined question of clinical relevance, e.g. is fluoride varnish effective in preventing dental caries? Check to see whether a systematic review on this topic has already been carried out. If so, is it up to date?
Draft the protocol for the review	This should be very clear on how the review will be conducted and should clearly describe the: • research question • search strategy • inclusion and exclusion criteria for studies • protocol for data extraction • approach to the statistical analysis of the data.
The search strategy	This is likely to be in several parts: • **Formal review** of the published literature. Help should be sought from an experienced librarian/information technologist to formulate the search strategy. This will need to define the bibliographic databases to be searched, e.g. Medline, EMBASE, CINAHL, and will vary according to the question being researched. The keywords and combination of keywords for the search will need to be agreed. The publication time frame for included studies will need to be defined, as will the languages of the studies to be included – either restricted to English or more usefully to include all languages. • **Hand search.** This involves screening the index pages of relevant journals to identify relevant studies that might not have been identified by the formal electronic search. Although called a hand search, these days this is likely to be conducted by looking at the index pages of the online version of relevant journals. • **Reference list/bibliography search**. The reference lists of relevant studies identified earlier are read to identify any studies not picked up in the original review. • **Grey literature** – this describes data that has not been formally published and may include data held by product manufacturers, data on websites, or data held by academics that has not been formally published. • **Specific call for information**. On occasion researchers conducting a systematic review will set up a website to which data may be submitted.
Identification of relevant studies	Following the search, the titles and abstracts of studies selected are screened to identify possible relevant studies – many of the studies identified by the searches will not meet the inclusion criteria. For example, in a systematic review of the effects of fluoride varnish, studies that were not in the form of a randomized controlled trial would be excluded.
Data extraction	Data from the studies identified as relevant are extracted and entered on a specifically designed database. So in the case of the systematic review on the clinical effectiveness of fluoride varnish, the magnitude of the caries increment in test and control groups would be noted, together with other relevant information, such as whether this was in primary or permanent teeth, the duration of the study, the frequency of the varnish application, the number of participants in the study.
Data analysis – **meta-analysis**	Provided that there are sufficient studies, using the same outcome measure, the outcome measure can be combined via an advanced statistical technique called a **meta-analysis**. This gives an overall idea of the effectiveness of the intervention being reviewed, and is reported using a **forest plot** (Figure 17.1). A major consideration is the heterogeneity of the studies to be included in the meta-analysis. Heterogeneity is said to exist where the variation in the estimates of the treatment effects reported by individual studies to be included in the systematic review is greater than would have been expected by chance. When a meta-analysis is not possible, a narrative review may be presented. Here the results are described in words, without a formal statistical estimate of the combined effects.
Reporting	Guidance on how to report a systematic review is provided by the PRISMA statement (Figure 17.2). This comprises a 27-statement checklist and a 4-phase flow diagram (www.prisma-statement.org/). **PRISMA** stands for **Preferred Reporting Items for Systematic reviews and Meta-Analyses**.

18 Evidence-based dentistry and clinical guidelines

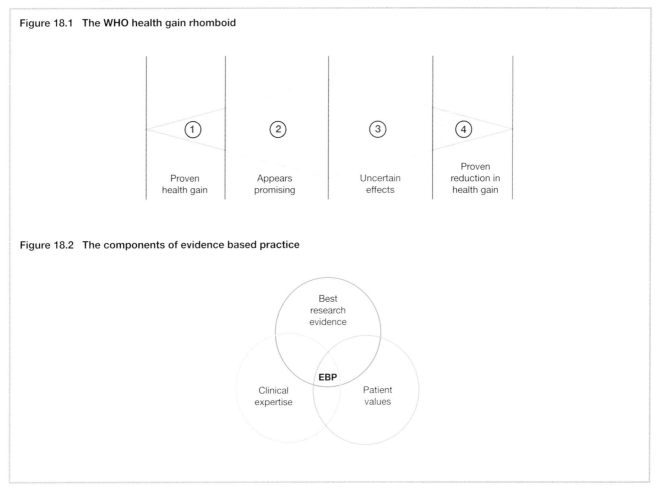

Figure 18.1 The WHO health gain rhomboid

① Proven health gain
② Appears promising
③ Uncertain effects
④ Proven reduction in health gain

Figure 18.2 The components of evidence based practice

Best research evidence

Clinical expertise

EBP

Patient values

Evidence-based practice

In 1972 Professor Archie Cochrane, who is now regarded as the 'father' of the evidence-based healthcare movement, published a document called 'Effectiveness and efficiency – random reflections on health services'. The basic tenet of Cochrane's observations was that in providing healthcare, efforts should be made to encourage the use of practices and procedures that have been shown by scientific study to provide a positive health gain. At the same time, interventions that are of no benefit or indeed that are harmful should not be used.

In 1996, Sackett and colleagues defined evidence-based practice as:

The conscientious, explicit and judicious use of current best evidence in making decisions about the care of individual patients. The practice of evidence-based medicine means integrating individual clinical expertise with the best available external clinical evidence from systematic research.

Evidence-based dentistry

By inference, evidence-based dentistry can be defined as follows:

Evidence-based dentistry is the practice of dentistry that integrates the best available evidence with clinical experience and patient preference in making clinical decisions.

The health gain rhomboid (Figure 18.1) categorizes treatments and procedures into one of four categories. The argument is that many treatments currently provided fall into categories 2 and 3, where their benefits are either promising or uncertain – but they have not been proven to be the most effective and efficient way to provide care. The aim of evidence-based practice is to deliver more and more treatments that are categorized in category 1; that is, they have been shown by scientific study to result in positive health gain. Procedures that result in harm to patients (category 4) should not be provided. While this seems obvious, there are numerous examples in the healthcare literature of procedures that continued to be provided, even after they had been proven to be ineffective, or even worse to be harmful.

In its guidance to members of the dental team, the General Dental Council requires the provision of quality care based on up-to-date evidence.

The Cochrane Collaboration

The Cochrane Collaboration (named in honour of Archie Cochrane) is an independent global network of researchers, clinicians, patients and individuals interested in healthcare whose mission is to promote evidence-informed health decision making by producing high-quality, relevant, accessible, systematic reviews and other synthesized research evidence.

Dental Public Health at a Glance, First Edition. Ivor G. Chestnutt.
© 2016 John Wiley & Sons, Ltd. Published 2016 by John Wiley & Sons, Ltd.

The most tangible aspect of the Cochrane Collaboration is the Cochrane Library (www.cochranelibrary.com). This contains over 200 systematic reviews of relevance to dental and oral health.

Clinical guidelines

Given the vast number of research studies published in any week, month or year, it is impossible for a busy clinician to keep up to date by reading and making sense of the original research articles. This is complicated by the fact that the articles will often have conflicting or equivocal results. Clinical guidelines have been developed to help overcome this problem.

Clinical guidelines attempt to synthesize the current evidence base in a format that can be read by healthcare providers. Used in conjunction with the clinician's personal experience and expertise and the patient's preferences, the hope is that the guidelines will inform evidence-based decisions and choices of treatment (Figure 18.2).

Levels of evidence

Guidelines often grade the level of evidence. This indicates where on the hierarchy of evidence (Table 11.1) the source of the guidance originates. For example, is it high-level evidence derived from a systematic review and meta-analysis, or is it merely expert opinion, adopted in the absence of robust evidence from formal research studies. An example of evidence statements and grades of recommendations as used by the Scottish Intercollegiate Guidelines Network (SIGN) is shown in Table 18.1.

Guideline producers

National Institute for Health and Care Excellence (NICE)

The National Institute for Health and Care Excellence (NICE) (www.nice.org.uk) is a non-departmental public body, which, while accountable to the Department of Health in England, is independent of government. The aims of NICE are to improve outcomes for people using the NHS and other public health and social care services. The functions of NICE include:
• producing evidence-based guidance and advice for health, public health and social care practitioners
• developing quality standards and performance metrics for those providing and commissioning health, public health and social care services
• providing a range of informational services for commissioners, practitioners and managers across the spectrum of health and social care.

NICE has produced guidelines of relevance to both clinical and dental public health practice (Table 18.2).

Scottish Intercollegiate Guidelines Network (SIGN)

The Scottish Intercollegiate Guidelines Network (SIGN), part of Healthcare Improvement Scotland, has produced guidelines of relevance to dentistry (Table 18.2).

Specialist societies

A number of specialist dental societies have produced guidelines of relevance to clinical practice with their area of interest (Table 18.2).

Table 18.1 Evidence statements and grades of recommendations as used by the Scottish Intercollegiate Guidelines Network (SIGN)

Levels of evidence

1^{++}	High-quality meta-analyses, systematic reviews of randomized controlled trials (RCTs) or RCTs with a very low risk of bias
1^{+}	Well-conducted meta-analyses, systematic reviews or RCTs with a low risk of bias
1^{-}	Meta-analyses, systematic reviews or RCTs with a high risk of bias
2^{++}	High-quality systematic reviews of case-control or cohort studies High-quality case-control or cohort studies with a very low risk of confounding or bias and a high probability that the relationship is causal
2^{+}	Well-conducted case-control or cohort studies with a low risk of confounding or bias and a moderate probability that the relationship is causal
2^{-}	Case-control or cohort studies with a high risk of confounding or bias and a significant risk that the relationship is not causal
3	Non-analytical studies, e.g. case reports, case series
4	Expert opinion

Grades of recommendation

Note: The grade of recommendation relates to the strength of the evidence on which the recommendation is based. It does not reflect the clinical importance of the recommendation.

A	At least one meta-analysis, systematic review or RCT rated as 1^{++} and directly applicable to the target population; *or* A body of evidence consisting principally of studies rated as 1^{+}, directly applicable to the target population and demonstrating overall consistency of results
B	A body of evidence including studies rated as 2^{++}, directly applicable to the target population and demonstrating overall consistency of results; *or* Extrapolated evidence from studies rated as 1^{++} or 1^{+}
C	A body of evidence including studies rated as 2^{+}, directly applicable to the target population and demonstrating overall consistency of results; *or* Extrapolated evidence from studies rated as 2^{++}
D	Evidence level 3 or 4; *or* Extrapolated evidence from studies rated as 2^{+}

Good practice points

✓	Recommended best practice based on the clinical experience of the guideline development group

Source: *SIGN 2014. Reproduced with permission from Scottish Intercollegiate Guidelines Network (SIGN).*

Table 18.2 Examples of clinical guidelines of relevance to dentistry

Guideline producer	Guideline title
British Orthodontic Society	A Guideline for the Extraction of First Permanent Molars in Children
British Society of Periodontology	Guidelines for Periodontal Screening and Management of Children and Adolescents under 18 Years of Age
National Institute for Health and Care Excellence (NICE)	Dental Recall
National Institute for Health and Care Excellence (NICE)	Guidance on the Extraction of Wisdom Teeth
National Institute for Health and Care Excellence (NICE)	Oral Health: Approaches for Local Authorities and Their Partners to Improve the Oral Health of Their Communities
National Institute for Health and Care Excellence (NICE)	Oral Health for Adults in Care Homes
National Institute for Health and Care Excellence (NICE)	Oral Health Promotion for Dental Teams
Scottish Intercollegiate Guidelines Network	Dental Interventions to Prevent Caries in Children

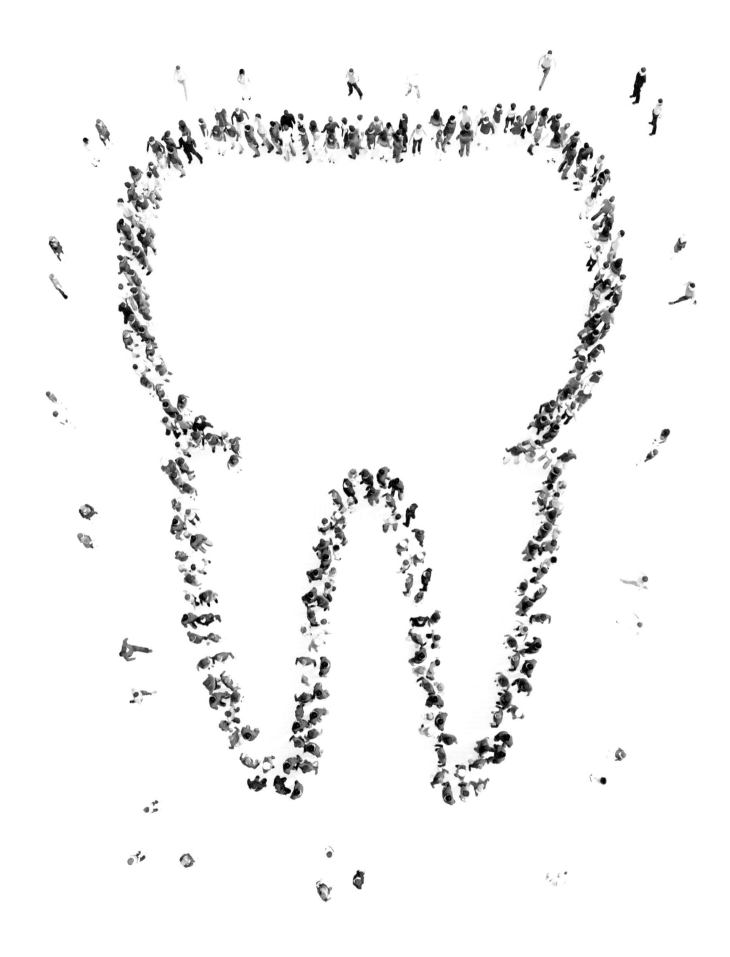

Oral health promotion

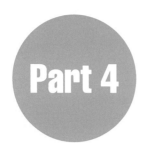

Part 4

Chapters

19 Inequalities in oral health

Figure 19.1   dmft at age 5 years by quintile of deprivation (Wales 2011–12)

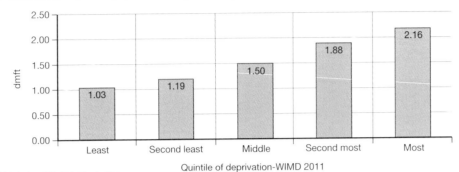

WIMD = Welsh Index of Multiple Deprivation

Figure 19.2   The distribution of dental caries in 5-year-old children (Wales 2011–12)

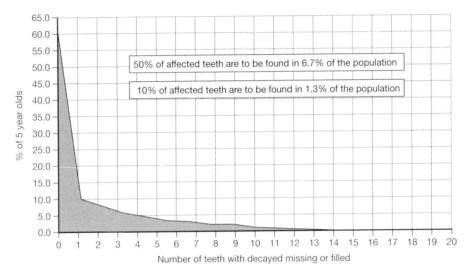

Figure 19.3   Diagrammatic representation of desirable and undesirable changes in the prevalence of disease by deprivation category following implementation of an oral health improvement programme

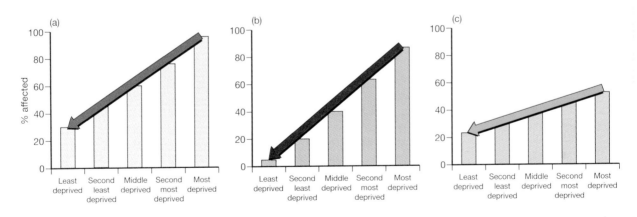

Diagrammatic representation of how oral health improvement programmes may affect health inequalities.

(a) Situation where disease prevalence is directly proportional to deprivation status (purple line)
(b) Represents the inequality gradient where implementation of an oral health improvement programme has disproportionately advantaged the least deprived - thereby widening the gap between least and most deprived - an undesirable consequence (red line)
(c) Represents the situation where an oral health improvement programme has favoured the most deprived quintiles thereby reducing oral health inequalities - a desired consequence (green line)

Dental Public Health at a Glance, First Edition. Ivor G. Chestnutt.
© 2016 John Wiley & Sons, Ltd. Published 2016 by John Wiley & Sons, Ltd.

The determinants of health were described in Chapter 2 and the significant gains in oral health observed in the United Kingdom in both children and adults over the past three decades were discussed in Chapter 9. However, the improvements in oral health have not been equally distributed across the population. In common with most lifestyle-influenced diseases, oral diseases are heavily influenced by social and economic status.

Measuring social and economic status

Social class

The concept of classifying the population based on social and economic status dates back to the 1850s. By the early twentieth century a measure of social class based on the occupation of the head of the household had been devised by the Registrar General's Office in the United Kingdom. This worked well for the first eight decades of the twentieth century. However, as working patterns and family structures changed, the occupational status of one individual in a household increasingly failed to reflect the growing number of families where two adults worked or where there was just one adult.

Area-based measures of deprivation

The limitations of social class as a measure of deprivation have led to the development of area-based measures. These relate not to an individual family but to the neighbourhood in which the family lives – an area that includes about 1500 people. This is called a Lower Layer Super Output Area (LLSOA). There are 32,844 LLSOAs in England and 1909 in Wales. For each LLSOA seven domains are measured (Table 19.1). These can be employed either separately or in combination to give a measure of relative deprivation (i.e. how deprived one locality is in relation to another). Using a patient's postcode, it is possible to determine the relative deprivation of where they live.

There are Indices of Multiple Deprivation for England, Scotland and Wales. To examine how disease prevalence relates to deprivation, it is possible to segment (divide up) the population into equal fifths (quintiles), sevenths (septiles) or tenths (deciles). As an example, Figure 19.1 shows how dental caries varies according to quintile of deprivation in Welsh 5-year-olds.

Reports on deprivation and health

There have been several prominent reports on the relationship between deprivation and health. The Black Report, published in 1980, is regarded as the seminal document to highlight inequalities in health across the social divide. The most recent report, *Fair Society, Healthy Lives* or the Marmot Report, published in 2010, set a number of indicators of the social determinants of health, health outcomes and social inequality and recommended actions to address health inequalities (Table 19.2).

Table 19.1 The domains that contribute to the Index of Multiple Deprivation

- Income
- Employment
- Health
- Education, skills and training
- Barriers to housing and services

Table 19.2 Marmot Indicators 2014 – actions to address health inequalities based on the Marmot Review (2010)

A Give every child the best start in life
B Enable all children, young people and adults to maximize their capabilities and have control over their lives
C Create fair employment and good work for all
D Ensure a healthy standard of living for all
E Create and develop healthy and sustainable places and communities
F Strengthen the role and impact of ill-health prevention

Inequalities in oral health

Children

Figure 5.5 demonstrates how the distribution of dental caries in populations has changed from being normally distributed to a skewed distribution where the disease is concentrated in fewer individuals, those from more deprived backgrounds. The distribution of dental caries in Welsh 5-year-olds is given in Figure 19.2. This demonstrates that just under 60% are caries free and that the disease is confined to 40% of the population. This distribution shows the 'high-risk' tail to the distribution, with 10% of carious teeth concentrated in just 1.3% of the population.

Adults

Demonstrating the impact of social and economic inequalities in adults is influenced by the measure of oral disease that is chosen and also the measure of social and economic deprivation. A recent analysis of the 2009 Adult Dental Health Survey concluded that oral health inequalities manifest in different ways in different age groups, representing age and cohort effects. So while there were no differences in the number of missing teeth by social class in younger adults, in older adults the least deprived had 4.5 fewer teeth missing than the most deprived.

In oral disease where the risk factors are heavily linked to social class, such as oral cancer, differences in disease prevalence across social divides are large. Not only is oral cancer more common in those from deprived backgrounds, adults from lower social class are more likely to present to a doctor or dentist when the cancer is at a more advanced stage and therefore with a poorer prognosis (Chapter 7).

Quantifying health inequalities

Figure 19.3 demonstrates the gradient in oral health across quintiles of deprivation (i.e. the population divided into equal fifths). A measure called the Slope Index of Inequality can be used to quantify the degree of difference across social classes. It represents the linear regression coefficient of the relation between the level of disease in each socio-economic category and the hierarchical ranking of each socio-economic category on the social scale (Figure 19.3a).

Addressing oral health inequalities

The aim of health improvement programmes should be to address inequalities in oral health. This requires careful consideration. The provision of a programme that is only taken up by those at the upper end and middle of the social spectrum has the potential to widen oral health inequalities (Figure 19.3b). Ideally, health improvement programmes should have a maximal effect on the most deprived, thereby flattening the inequality slope (Figure 19.3c). Strategic approaches to improving oral health are discussed further in Chapter 23.

20 Oral health education, oral health promotion and oral health improvement

Figure 20.1 Health Promotion - a combination of health education, prevention and health protection.
Source: *Data from Downie et al. 1990.*

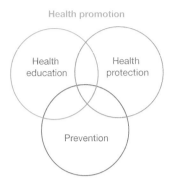

Figure 20.2 The concept of upstream and downstream approaches to oral health improvement

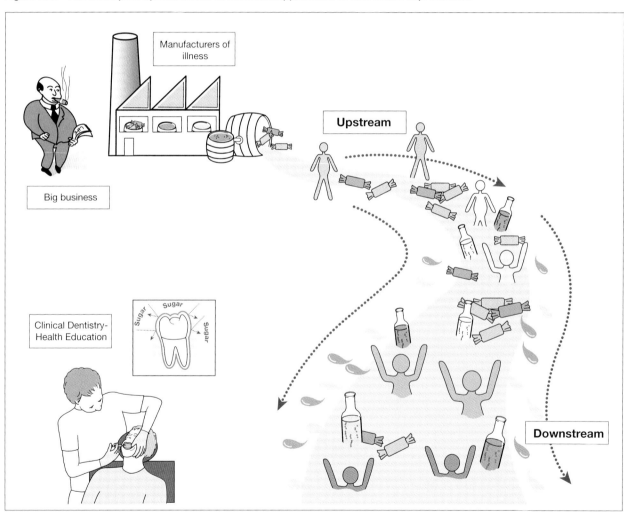

Preventing disease and improving health is one of the three key objectives of public health. The other two are *improving services* and *health protection* (the prevention of infectious disease and environmental hazards).

Health improvement requires a key understanding of the determinants of health (Chapter 2). Securing health involves action at different levels – the *individual, professional health and care services* and *society*. The balance between these aspects and where responsibility for preventing disease and securing health lies are frequently matters of debate. As an example, in the prevention of dental caries, should the responsibility lie with individuals who, by reducing the frequency of sugar consumption and brushing

Dental Public Health at a Glance, First Edition. Ivor G. Chestnutt.
© 2016 John Wiley & Sons, Ltd. Published 2016 by John Wiley & Sons, Ltd.

their teeth with a fluoride toothpaste, markedly reduce their caries risk, or should individuals be helped by the government imposing a tax on sugared drinks and implementing water fluoridation?

Health promotion is an all-encompassing concept that in addition to *health education* includes *health protection* and *prevention* (Figure 20.1).

Health education is the provision of information to individuals and populations on how to prevent disease and improve health.

Health protection comprises laws, regulations, policies and voluntary codes of practice aimed at preventing disease and enhancing health, for instance seat-belt laws or no-smoking policies.

Prevention includes patient-based interventions such as fissure sealants or application of fluoride varnish.

Approaches to health improvement

Oral health education

There are six key messages in securing oral health and preventing dental disease (Table 20.1). It is important that individuals understand and act on these messages. Dental professionals have an important role to play in delivering these messages on a one-to-one basis at the chairside. This is one of the few opportunities when individuals can have the messages tailored to their own particular needs and circumstances.

Limitations of oral health education

While oral health education is important on a one-to-one basis, it has a number of limitations:

- **Knowledge, attitudes, behaviour:** Changes in knowledge do not necessarily lead to changes in behaviour. Education may enhance knowledge and alter an individual's attitude and desire to live more healthily. However, this does not mean that they will necessarily change their behaviour. So an individual may know that smoking is detrimental to their periodontal health and may want to stop smoking, but the effort involved plus the addiction to nicotine may prevent them from changing their behaviour and stopping smoking.
- **Short-term improvements:** even if an individual manages to change their behaviour, this is often short lived – New Year's resolutions are a typical example of how well-intentioned actions to engage in health behaviours may not last more than a few days or weeks.
- **Personal circumstances may preclude action:** eating a diet rich in fruit and vegetables – the 5-a-day message – may be difficult for a family from a poor background where cost, access and cooking skills may well inhibit them from taking up this recommendation.
- **Medical model outdated:** often health promotion messages promote health only in terms of the absence of disease, and the wider dimensions of health are ignored.
- **Negative – disease focused, victim blaming:** many health education messages are negative, focusing on what people should not do rather than on what they should.

Table 20.1 The key messages for oral health education

- **Diet:** reduce both the amount and frequency of intake of sugar-containing food and drink – 'Eat less sugar and eat sugar less often'
- **Tooth brushing:** clean your teeth thoroughly twice every day with a fluoride toothpaste
- **Dental attendance:** have a regular oral examination at a time interval recommended by your dentist, based on your risk of oral disease
- **Mouthguards:** Always wear a custom-made mouthguard when participating in contact sports
- **Tobacco:** do not smoke tobacco or use tobacco in any other form
- **Alcohol:** consume alcohol in moderation and keep to the recommended weekly limits. Have alcohol-free days each week and do not binge drink

- **Directive:** many health education messages are dictatorial and fail to recognize people's individual life circumstances.
- **Potential to widen inequalities in health:** inappropriately applied health education that is only acted on by the least deprived has the potential to widen oral health inequalities (Figure 19.3).
- **Conflicting messages:** contradictory messages, often promoted by the media who like controversial stories, can confuse the public and undo years of good work by disrupting public understanding of the evidence.
- **Limited evidence of benefit in group settings:** although talks to parents and children in schools have traditionally fulfilled a role otherwise undertaken by dental educators, in the absence of an intervention involving the provision of fluoride there is little evidence that classroom health education is effective.

The Ottawa Charter

Health education was the traditional approach to improving health. It has an important role on a one-to-one basis, but has limited potential on a population basis. Probably the most influential development in the field of health improvement was the production of the Ottawa Charter in 1986. This statement was produced by the World Health Organization following the first International Conference on Health Promotion, meeting in Ottawa, Canada. The principles espoused by the charter are shown in Table 20.2. It has been extremely influential over the past 30 years in how governments and health providers think of health promotion.

The Ottawa Charter recognized that the potential to improve health on a population basis was limited by the then prevailing health education approach. It stressed the need to work at a 'higher level' and tackle the wider determinants of health by addressing issues at the level of personal autonomy, communities and public policy.

Upstream and downstream health promotion

These terms arise from the concepts in the Ottawa Charter. **Upstream** refers to actions taken at a policy level to prevent disease and promote health. **Downstream** actions are those carried out at an individual level. Because they have greater potential to reach many more people and do not require them to take any action individually, upstream actions are potentially more effective than downstream actions. Policies directed at controlling the production and availability of sugared sweets and drinks are likely to be more effective than actions by a dentist advising patients on dietary restriction of sugar (Figure 20.2).

Table 20.2 The principles of the Ottawa Charter

- **Promoting health through public policy:** this recognizes that it is necessary to reach beyond the health sector to address the determinants of health fully. Restriction on the sale of tobacco and alcohol to children is an example of a health-protecting public policy.
- **Creating a supportive environment:** this recognizes the socio-geographical and environmental aspects of promoting health. Banning smoking in public places is an example of how the environment in pubs and clubs has been changed to protect bar workers from the dangers of passive smoking (breathing someone else's tobacco smoke).
- **Developing personal skills:** this involves helping individuals to develop the skills necessary to keep themselves and their family healthy. An example would be teaching young parents how to prepare and cook fresh fruit and vegetables to encourage healthy eating and reduce reliance on unhealthy pre-prepared and convenience foods.
- **Strengthening community action:** this encourages local communities to come together to pool resources and knowledge to promote health – establishment of local sports clubs would encourage physical exercise, for example.

21 **Considerations in promoting oral health**

Figure 21.1 **Common-risk factor approach.** Source: *Watt 2005. Reproduced with permission from World Health Organisation. Originally adapted from Sheiham and Watt 2000 with permission from John Wiley & Sons.*

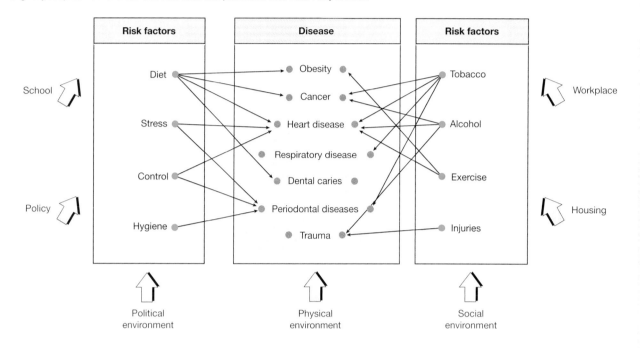

Figure 21.2 **An outcome model for health promotion.** Source: *Nutbeam 1998. Reproduced with permission from Oxford University Press.*

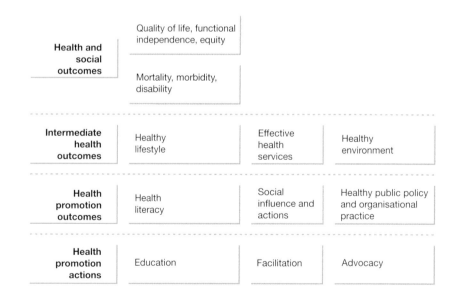

Tackling risk factors

Addressing risk factors for disease can be approached from two perspectives: a disease-centred approach and a common risk factor approach.

Disease-centred approach

In this outdated approach, the risk factor(s) for an individual disease are considered solely in relation to that one disease. This has the potential to lead to conflicting advice being given and failure to maximize the impact of preventive activities. As an example, foods like cheese and potato crisps are not cariogenic and so if health educators were to approach the prevention of dental caries purely from a dental perspective, the message that cheese is acceptable as a snack between meals might be acceptable and thus promoted. However, those concerned with the prevention of obesity and cardiovascular disease would be likely to be less happy to promote these foods as a snack.

Common risk factor approach

Here the focus is not on a single disease but rather, as the name implies, on the risk factors. This approach recognizes that one risk factor can contribute to more than one disease. Helping people stop smoking not only reduces the risk of developing cardiovascular disease, but oral cancer, periodontal attachment loss and any of the many other diseases in which tobacco use increases disease risk. A diagrammatic representation of the common risk factor approach is presented in Figure 21.1. This shows how alcohol is a risk factor for cancers, heart disease and trauma.

The common risk factor approach reduces the danger of individuals being given conflicting advice and also maximizes the health gain from adopting the advice given. Dental public health practitioners should look for opportunities to ensure that messages relevant to oral health are given when general health promotion campaigns are being planned. For example, in smoking-cessation campaigns it is important to include the effects of smoking on oral health as well as general health.

Settings approach to health promotion

In this context a **setting** is a place or environment where groups of similar individuals meet or gather. Examples are schools, hospitals and workplaces. Sometimes health promotion campaigns and actions are based around settings. The concept of '**health-promoting schools**' has been used to ensure that schools and education authorities facilitate healthy behaviours and offer appropriate messages to children. This might involve environmental changes such as banning vending machines selling sugared drinks, the provision of water to drink in class and the promotion of fruit-only tuck shops. Educational activities would focus on health issues relevant to children and young people, such as advice on smoking, alcohol, bullying and sexual health issues.

The role of the media and technology in promoting health

Traditional media

Newspaper, magazine, billboard, radio and television advertising is occasionally used to promote health education messages. Graphic images and messages associated with smoking or the effects of not wearing a seat belt are recent examples. These are effective in raising awareness. However, advertising is expensive and health bodies usually do not have an advertising budget to compete with companies advertising sugar-rich foods and drinks.

Advertisements promoting cigarettes have been severely curtailed in the past two decades, including a ban on the sponsorship of sporting events by tobacco companies. Similarly, restrictions have been implemented on advertising sugary foods and drinks during children's television programmes.

Social media

Social media – blogs, Twitter, Facebook, forums and message boards – are a new route whereby health improvement messages can be communicated and the opinions of stakeholders gathered. Patient and public involvement (PPI) in the design and delivery of health-promoting activities is important and increases engagement and potential take-up. Social media also provides a means of disseminating messages to groups whom it might otherwise be difficult to reach, such as teenagers.

Social marketing

Social marketing uses techniques from the world of marketing to influence behaviours that benefit individuals and communities for the greater social good (rather than marketing the use of goods or services). This technique has been employed successfully in Australia to encourage the use of sun-screening products by fair-skinned individuals exposed to the fierce Antipodean sun.

Evaluating oral health promotion

Health promotion is about giving people control over and the chance to improve their health, but it also involves complex social and political interventions: education, facilitation and advocacy. Like with all healthcare, it is important to ensure that health promotion activities are evidence based and achieve their desired outcome. This can be complex, given that the ultimate desired outcome – improved health, environmental or social conditions – may occur months, years or even decades after the intervention. An outcome model for health promotion is shown in Figure 21.2.

The following factors should be considered when evaluating a health promotion intervention:

- **Effectiveness:** whether the aims and objectives of the intervention have been met.
- **Appropriateness:** the relevance of the intervention to needs.
- **Acceptability:** the degree to which the intervention is acceptable and carried out in a sensitive manner.
- **Efficiency:** whether time, money and other resources devoted to the programme are well spent in relation to the benefits observed.
- **Equity:** whether the programme has been delivered in relation to needs and the capacity to benefit.

22 Behaviour change

Figure 22.1 The components of the health belief model. Source: *Rosenstock et al. 1994. Reproduced with permission from Springer Science + Business Media.*

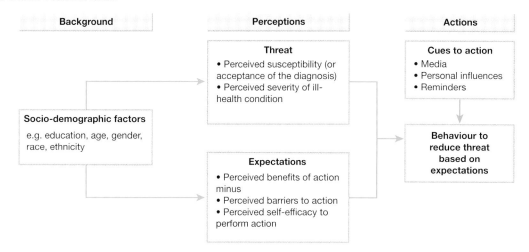

Figure 22.2 The theory of planned behaviour, which suggests that attitudes, beliefs and behavioural control are important antecedents to behaviour change (described by Ajzen) Source: *Ajzen 1991. Reproduced with permission from Elsevier.* **See box 22.1**

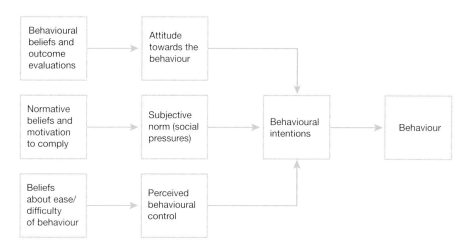

Box 22.1 The constructs underpinning the Theory of Planned Behaviour

The Theory of Planned Behaviour comprises six constructs that collectively represent a person's actual control over their behaviour:
1 **Attitudes** – the degree to which a person has a favourable or unfavourable evaluation of the behaviour of interest. It entails consideration of the outcomes of performing the behaviour.
2 **Behavioural intention** – the motivational factors that influence a given behaviour. where the stronger the intention to perform the behaviour, the more likely it is that the behaviour will be performed.
3 **Subjective norms** – the belief about whether most people approve or disapprove of the behaviour. It relates to a person's beliefs about whether peers and people of importance to the person think he or she should engage in the behaviour.
4 **Social norms** – the customary codes of behaviour in a group of people or larger cultural context. Social norms are considered normative, or standard, in a group of people.
5 **Perceived power** – the perceived presence of factors that may facilitate or impede performance of a behaviour. Perceived power contributes to a person's perceived behavioural control over each of those factors.
6 **Perceived behavioural control** – a person's perception of the ease or difficulty of performing the behaviour of interest. Perceived behavioural control varies across situations and actions, which results in a person having varying perceptions of behavioural control depending on the situation. This construct of the theory was added later, and created the shift from the Theory of Reasoned Action to the Theory of Planned Behaviour.

Dental Public Health at a Glance, First Edition. Ivor G. Chestnutt.
© 2016 John Wiley & Sons, Ltd. Published 2016 by John Wiley & Sons, Ltd.

The major dental diseases are heavily influenced by lifestyle and behavioural choices. If individuals can be persuaded to change their behaviour, then they can make healthy choices and avoid actions detrimental to good oral health. However, behaviour change is a complex process. Many theories of behaviour and behaviour change have been proposed and those of most relevance to oral health are outlined here.

Knowledge, attitudes, behaviour

Knowledge → Attitudes → Behaviour

The earliest theories of behaviour change arising in the early twentieth century assumed that educating people and changing attitudes would result in behaviour change. The simplistic assumption that providing or improving knowledge via education would be sufficient to change attitudes and hence lead to sustained behaviour change has been shown to be erroneous. Psychological theories arising in the mid-twentieth century recognized that behaviour change is complicated by beliefs, ways of thinking (cognition) and environmental and social factors.

Theories of behaviour change

Three of the most common models underpinning theories of behaviour change are the *Health Belief Model*, the *Theory of Planned Behaviour* and the *Trans-theoretical Model*.

Health Belief Model

The Health Belief Model was one of the earliest health belief models and was developed in the early 1950s by social scientists at the US Public Health Service in order to understand the failure of people to adopt disease-prevention strategies or take up screening tests for the early detection of disease (Figure 22.1). The model suggests that a person's likelihood of taking preventive action depends on the interaction of various beliefs:

• The perceived threat from the disease (based on the perceived susceptibility to the disease and the perceived severity or impact of the disease).

• The expectations associated with taking preventive action (based on the perceived barriers to taking action, alongside the perceived benefit of taking action in reducing the threat of a disease).

Theory of Planned Behaviour

The Theory of Planned Behaviour was adapted from an earlier model (the Theory of Reasoned Action). It suggests that people form positive or negative intentions to behave in a certain way on the basis of their *subjective norms*, their *perceived behavioural control* and their *attitude towards the behaviour*. This attitude is said to be based on their belief about the likely consequences of an action and their desire to achieve those outcomes (Figure 22.2 and Box 22.1).

Trans-theoretical Model

Developed by Prochaska and DiClemente in the late 1970s, this model assumes that behaviour change is evolutional in nature and occurs in stages of change through which individuals can progress. It holds that behaviours, especially habitual behaviours such as smoking, follow a series of steps through a cyclical process (Chapter 32, Figure 32.1).

NICE public health guidance on behaviour change

The National Institute of Health and Care Excellence (NICE) has issued public health guidance on behaviour change at both individual and population levels. Key findings in this guidance indicate that in promoting behaviour change it is important to facilitate the following:

• Make people aware of **outcome expectancies** and help them develop accurate knowledge about the health consequences of their behaviours.

• Emphasize the **personal relevance** of health behaviours.

• Promote **positive attitudes** and feelings towards the outcomes of behaviour change.

• Promote **self-efficacy** by enhancing people's belief in their ability to change.

• **Descriptive norms** – promote the visibility of positive health behaviours in people's reference groups; that is, the groups that they compare themselves to or aspire to.

• **Subjective norms** – enhance social approval for positive health behaviours in significant others and reference groups.

• Promote **personal and moral norms** – personal and moral commitments to behaviour change.

• Suggest **intention formation and concrete plans** – help people to form plans and goals for changing behaviours, over time and in specific contexts.

• **Behavioural contracts** – suggest that people share their plans and goals with others.

Locus of control

A concept that is closely related to people's health-related beliefs is their 'locus of control': the extent to which they broadly believe that their health is determined by events over which they have personal control (**an internal locus of control**) or events over which they have little or no control (**an external locus of control**).

Motivational interviewing

Motivational interviewing is a form of collaborative conversation that is designed to strengthen a person's own motivation and commitment to change. It is a person-centred style of counselling that attempts to address ambivalence about change. The process sets a specific change goal by examining the person's own reason for change.

The ethos is that in facilitating behaviour change, the idea is not to confront the person wanting to change but to motivate them. So rather than say 'Why don't you brush your teeth twice a day?' ask 'What do you think would be the benefits of brushing twice a day?'

The mnemonic **FRAMES** is designed to help remember specific aspects of motivational interviewing:

F – provide **f**eedback on behaviour

R – reinforce patient's **r**esponsibility for changing behaviour

A – offer **a**dvice about changing behaviour

M – discuss a **m**enu of options to change behaviour

E – express **e**mpathy for the patient

S – support the patient's **s**elf-efficacy (own belief in their ability to change)

It is the patient's task to say how and why they should change behaviour; the clinician's task is to elicit these arguments.

23 Strategies for improving oral health in populations

Figure 23.1 Approaches to tackling oral health improvement: (a) high-risk individuals, (b) whole population, (c) high-risk population, (d) proportionate universalism

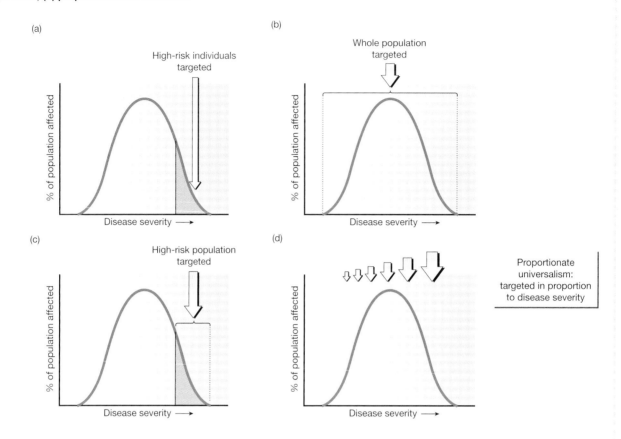

Figure 23.2 Example of an oral health improvement target. *Set in 2008 as part of the Child Poverty Reduction programme, the objective is by 2020, to reduce the prevalence of dental caries in the fifth most deprived quintile of the population to that experienced by the middle deprived quintile in 2008*

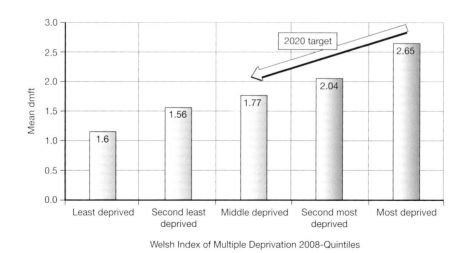

Set in 2008 as part of the Welsh Child Poverty Reduction Programme, the objective is by 2020, to reduce the prevalence of dental caries in the fifth most deprived quintile of the population to that experienced by the middle deprived quintile in 2008

Dental Public Health at a Glance, First Edition. Ivor G. Chestnutt.
© 2016 John Wiley & Sons, Ltd. Published 2016 by John Wiley & Sons, Ltd.

Improving population oral health can be approached in a number of ways

- High-risk individual approach
- Whole population approach
- Targeted population approach
- Proportionate universalism

High-risk individual approach

This approach to improving health involves the identification of those individuals who are at particular risk of disease and taking measures to reduce exposure to identified risk factors. This is the approach that is applied in clinical practice on a daily basis and it seeks to protect susceptible individuals (Figure 23.1a).

Example: A 6-year-old child attending a dental practice can be identified as at high risk for dental caries on the basis of already having decay in their primary dentition and the dentist's knowledge of the child's family and life circumstances. The clinician would then identify the child as being in need of additional preventive care and the provision of fissure sealants, fluoride varnish and dietary counselling would be appropriate.

Whole population approach

This approach is attributed to the thinking of Geoffrey Rose, who argued that it was necessary to consider not only the determinants of disease in individuals, but also the determinants of incidence rates in different populations. This approach seeks to control the causes of incidence. In relation to dental caries, it has been argued that targeting high-risk individuals while benefiting those identified neglects the fact that the majority of new carious lesions occur in lower-risk individuals, simply because there are many more of them.

Example: Advice to the whole population to 'brush your teeth twice a day with a fluoride-containing toothpaste' targets everyone and is held to have resulted in a massive shift in the distribution of dental decay in the population as a whole since the early 1970s (Figures 5.5 and 23.1b).

Targeted population approach

This approach to improving population oral health is a hybrid of the high-risk and whole population approaches. Here, the assessment of risk is not made on an individual basis, but on a population or locality basis. The correlation between dental caries and social and economic deprivation means that a much greater proportion of children resident in disadvantaged areas will experience dental decay. Population-based preventive efforts such as supervised school-based tooth-brushing programmes can be directed at these geographical localities.

Example: The Designed to Smile oral health improvement programme in Wales is an example of a targeted population approach. Here efforts are focused on areas of social and economic deprivation, in an attempt to improve oral health where disease is at its highest and by doing so address inequalities across the social spectrum (Figure 23.1c).

Proportionate universalism

Described by Marmot, this concept encourages an approach that, rather than targeting all available preventive resources at those at highest risk, proposes that preventive measures should be applied across the population in proportion to risk. This combines the advantages of all the other approaches described (Figure 23.1d).

The impact of preventive strategies on health inequalities

Setting strategies for populations with the intent of reducing inequalities in health needs careful consideration. A whole population approach, applied without appropriate care, has the potential to widen health inequalities (Figure 19.3). This can occur if the preventive activity is taken up by the least deprived to a greater extent than the most deprived – which is a highly likely scenario, given that the less deprived are better placed and probably more motivated to take advantage of health improvement initiatives.

Example: In the 1970s and 1980s, before the dominance of the topical effect of fluoride in preventing dental caries was realized, fluoride tablet and drop distribution schemes were popular as a population preventive measure, the thinking being that the fluoride would be taken up by the teeth during development. Issues of how fluoride works aside, these schemes had limited impact, as it was the motivated parents, whose children were at lower risk, who were most likely to adhere to the regime of giving the fluoride supplements to their children and to seek out further supplies. As a result, population-based fluoride supplement distribution schemes have long since been abandoned.

Targets in healthcare and health improvement

A target is a numerical goal often set as a policy objective. Currently there is much debate on the merits of setting targets in healthcare. Unless they are carefully chosen, there is an argument that they have the potential to skew clinical priorities. However, politicians favour targets as a simple means of assessing the success or otherwise of the National Health Service. Perhaps the best-known example of a healthcare target in the NHS at this time is that no one should have to wait for more than four hours before being seen in an Accident and Emergency department.

When developing health improvement strategies, it can be helpful to set a target. One such example was that set when the Designed to Smile programme was established in Wales in 2008. That stated that by 2020 the prevalence of dental decay in 5-year-olds in the most deprived quintile should have fallen to that present in the middle deprived quintile in 2008 (thereby reducing inequalities in oral health; Figure 23.2).

Assessing disease risk

In the past three decades a great deal of research has been carried out to develop risk assessment tools to determine individual susceptibility to developing oral disease. The multifactorial nature of dental caries, periodontal disease and oral cancer means that there has been limited success in the development of a single diagnostic risk assessment test. In assessing dental caries risk, the two most significant risk indicators for future caries development in children have been previous experience of dental caries and the subjective opinion of the treating clinician.

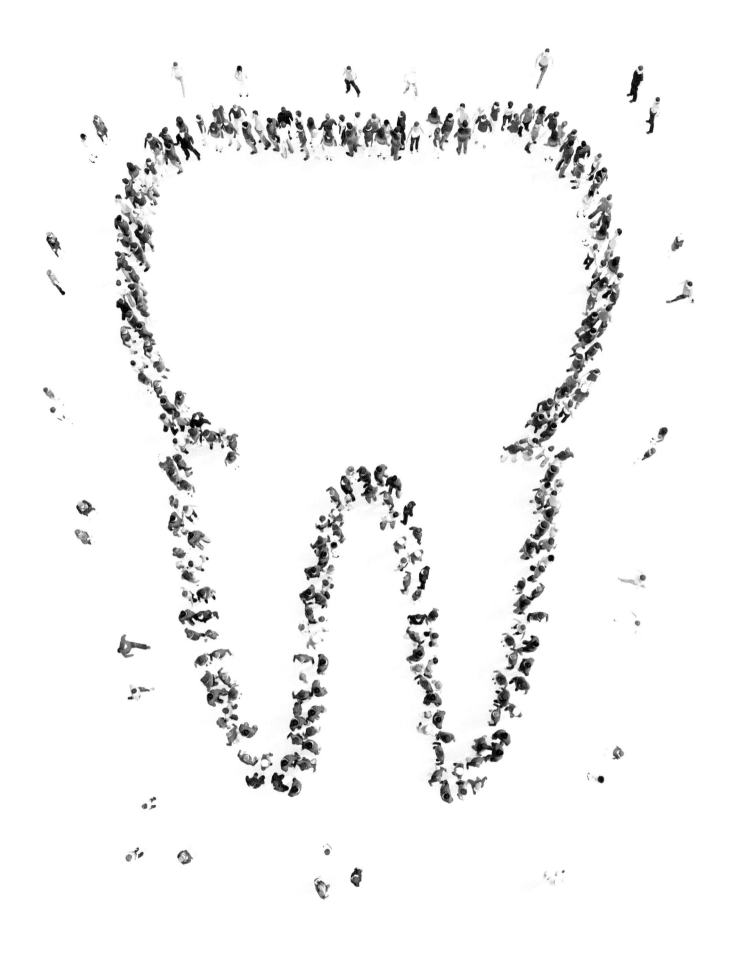

Fluoride and oral health

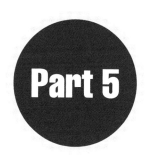

Part 5

Chapters

24 Strategies for the delivery of fluoride in the prevention of dental caries

Figure 24.1   Fluoride in the plaque biofilm inhibits demineralisation and promotes remineralisation of the hydroxyapatite crystals that form the tooth enamel

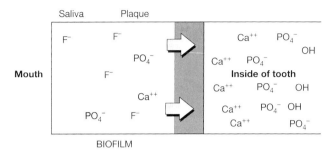

Figure 24.2a   Fluoride concentration in biofilm - sufficient to have caries protective effect

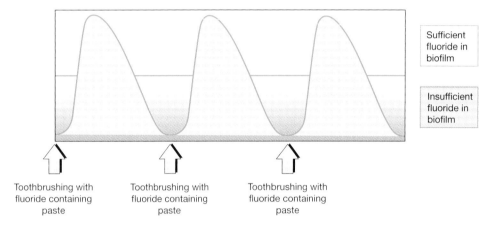

Figure 24.2b   Fluoride concentration in biofilm - exposure insufficient to have a clinically beneficial effect

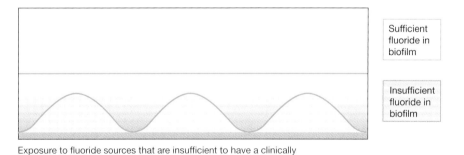

Exposure to fluoride sources that are insufficient to have a clinically beneficial effect, e.g. toothpaste containing <1000 ppm F

Figure 24.3   Fluoride strategies

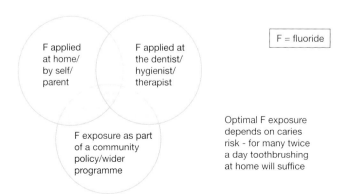

How fluoride acts to prevent dental caries

To understand how fluoride can be used to prevent dental caries at a population level, it is necessary to review how fluoride works to prevent dental decay at an anatomical and biochemical level. Dental enamel is composed in the main of calcium and phosphate ions in a crystalline structure called hydroxyapatite. When the pH of the fluid within the plaque biofilm immediately adjacent to the tooth falls as a result of bacterial acids derived from the fermentation of dietary carbohydrates, calcium and phosphate ions are lost from the enamel crystals. Initially this happens below the surface in the depths of the enamel prisms, as the acid acts on the porous areas between the enamel prisms that are vulnerable to acid attack. The earliest visible sign of this process is a 'white spot' enamel lesion. Unchecked, this process proceeds until a cavity develops.

From the discovery of the anticariogenic potential of fluoride in the early twentieth century until the beginning of the 1980s, it was thought that the main mechanism of action of fluoride in the prevention of dental caries depended on its incorporation into the dental enamel during tooth development pre-eruption – the **systemic effect**. The substitution of the hydroxyl ions in the hydroxyapatite crystals with a fluoride ion results in fluorapatite. This is more resistant to breakdown when subject to attack by acids derived from the fermentation of sugar by cariogenic bacteria once the tooth erupts into the mouth.

However, it is now understood that while the systemic effect occurs, the main mechanism of action of fluoride is its effect in encouraging the net uptake of calcium and fluoride ions at the tooth surface post-eruption – the **topical effect**. The presence of fluoride ions in the plaque fluid or biofilm that covers the tooth surface acts to drive calcium and phosphate into the tooth – **remineralization** (Figure 24.1). Fluoride works to inhibit demineralization at the crystal surfaces inside the tooth and to enhance the remineralization at the crystal surfaces – the resulting remineralized layer is very resistant to subsequent acid attack.

Research has also shown that fluoride inhibits sugar metabolism by plaque bacteria, but this effect is likely to be of limited clinical significance. It is the topical effect that is most important.

Fluoride in the plaque biofilm

In order that fluoride can exert this topical effect, it needs to be present in the plaque biofilm at a sufficient level to facilitate remineralization and prevent demineralization. Regular exposure to fluoride at recurring intervals helps maintain a level of fluoride that is sufficiently high to have an anticariogenic or cariostatic effect (Figure 24.2a). Exposure to sources of fluoride that contain an insufficiently high concentration of fluoride or that are used insufficiently frequently results in a lack of caries protection (Figure 24.2b).

Mechanisms for delivering fluoride

Fluoride can be made available in three main ways: via vehicles that patients apply themselves; via agents applied by dental professionals; via community fluoridation schemes (Table 24.1).

Developing a fluoride strategy

Public health professionals, in designing strategies to protect and improve oral health, need to think about how different sources of

Table 24.1 Mechanisms for the delivery of fluoride as a caries-preventive agent

Applied by patient or their parent	Applied by a dental professional: dentist, hygienist or therapist (in the UK dental nurses who have undergone additional training can apply fluoride varnish)	Community fluoridation schemes
Toothpaste (dentifrices)	Varnish	Water
Mouthwash	Gels	Milk
Tablets and drops	Indirectly via restorative materials, e.g. glass ionomer cements	Salt

Note: *Evidence for the effectiveness of these different ways of delivering fluoride is discussed in Chapters 25–27.*

fluoride may combine to provide a level of protection relative to the risk of different population groups, to provide optimal exposure to fluoride for each individual in the population (Figure 24.3). This is dictated by caries risk.

For those who maintain good oral hygiene and who do not consume a diet that exposes them to fermentable carbohydrates in excess quantity or frequency, twice-daily brushing with a toothpaste that contains at least 1000 parts per million (ppm) fluoride will provide adequate exposure to fluoride. For those at greater risk of dental caries, additional fluoride supplementation in the form of fluoride mouthwashes (e.g. when wearing a fixed orthodontic appliance) or fluoride varnish applied by a member of the dental team (e.g. when multiple early caries lesions are detected during a clinical examination) may be required. If using a fluoride mouthwash, this should be used at different times of the day to tooth brushing to maintain a sufficient background level of fluoride in the biofilm.

Community fluoridation schemes have one major advantage over professionally or self-applied fluoride – they do not require any active involvement on the part of the individual at risk. This is fortuitous, as those at greatest risk of dental caries (lower social and economic classes) are also those least likely to take active steps to use fluoride regularly or to maintain a low-sugar diet.

Exposure to excess fluoride and dental fluorosis

Exposure to excess fluoride during the period of tooth formation risks interfering with the secretion and maturation of the dental enamel on the tooth crown. Excess levels of fluoride in the body at this time can disrupt the functioning of ameloblasts. As a result, on eruption teeth can have defects in the enamel structure – **fluorosis**. These range from mild white spots (hypomineralization), which are barely noticeable unless the tooth is dried and examined carefully, to structural defects in the enamel, which appear as brownish yellow pits (hypoplasia). Fluorosis can be distinguished from other defects of dental enamel as it has a symmetrical distribution about the midline.

25 Toothpaste

Table 25.1 Factors affecting the clinical effectiveness of toothpaste in preventing dental caries

Factor	Notes
Presence of fluoride Fluoride containing toothpaste vs non-fluoride paste	A systematic review of 70 studies (involving 42300 children) reported that when tested against a non-fluoride control, fluoride toothpaste demonstrated a pooled prevented fraction of 24% DMFS. The 95% confidence interval was 21–28% with P < 0.0001. This means that fluoride toothpaste will reduce caries experience by about one quarter. A number needed to treat analysis showed that 1.6 children need to brush with a fluoride toothpaste to prevent one DMFS in populations with a caries increment of 2.6 DMFS per year. In populations with a caries increment of 1.1 DMFS per year, 3.7 children need to brush to avoid one DMFS.
Fluoride concentration	A systematic review demonstrated that toothpastes containing a fluoride concentration of 550 parts per million (ppm) F were no more effective than a non-fluoride control. Toothpastes between 1000 and 1250 ppm F have a prevented fraction of 23%, while those containing between 2400 and 2800 ppm F prevented 36% more caries that the non-fluoride control.
Volume of toothpaste	The amount of toothpaste used by young children should be carefully controlled to avoid excess exposure to fluoride during the period of tooth formation and thereby reduce the risk of dental fluorosis. Young children should not be allowed to eat toothpaste or lick the tube. Like all medicines, toothpaste should be stored safely out of the reach of children. **Children aged up to 3 years** Use no more than a thin smear of toothpaste (a thin film of paste covering less than three-quarters of the brush). The toothpaste should contain no less than 1000 ppm F. **Children aged 3–6 years** Use a pea-sized amount of toothpaste containing 1350–1500 ppm F.
Method of rinsing	In clinical trials where children were asked how they rinsed their mouth after brushing, those who rinsed from a beaker had more caries than those who rinsed using lesser quantities of water. For maximal effect it is important not to rinse after brushing, as this washes the fluoride down the sink and the topical effect is lost. However, it is important that children do not swallow toothpaste, especially in the period when the teeth are developing. Hence the message: **SPIT – DON'T RINSE**.
Frequency of tooth brushing	Those who brush at least twice a day experience significantly less caries than those who brush once a day or less.
Time spent brushing	There is no good evidence on the optimal time to spend brushing. Spending sufficient time to remove plaque and biofilm from difficult-to-reach areas seems sensible. Two minutes is often suggested as the optimum time.
Morning or night-time brushing	Brushing last thing at night and not eating or drinking afterwards is important in ensuring that a good intraoral fluoride reservoir is available overnight.
Brush before or after breakfast	There is a concern that brushing immediately after eating, especially if an acidic drink has been consumed, risks removing calcium and phosphate from the fluid adjacent to the tooth surface. The alternative view is that not brushing after breakfast leaves the oral cavity deficient in fluoride.
Starting tooth brushing	Parents should be encouraged to brush their child's teeth with a smear of toothpaste containing 1000 ppm F from when the teeth first erupt.
Powered vs manual toothbrush	There is evidence of difference in the effectiveness of powered vs manual tooth brushing. However, both are likely to be equally effective in increasing the concentration of intraoral fluoride.

Dental Public Health at a Glance, First Edition. Ivor G. Chestnutt.
© 2016 John Wiley & Sons, Ltd. Published 2016 by John Wiley & Sons, Ltd.

History

Powders and potions for cleaning the teeth date back to ancient civilizations. Over the centuries many different ingredients have been used, such as soot, chalk, crushed egg shells and tree bark. These medicaments had no therapeutic effect other than perhaps freshening the mouth if combined with herbs and oils.

Modern toothpastes contain a combination of 'active ingredients' aimed at simultaneously combating a range of oral conditions and in recent years have focused on the cosmetic as well as the therapeutic benefits of toothpaste.

Fluoride-containing toothpaste

The widespread availability of fluoride-containing toothpaste from the 1970s onwards is thought to have played a major role in the improvement in oral health seen in most developed countries. Various forms of fluoride have been incorporated into toothpaste over the years. The most common formulations contain either sodium fluoride, sodium monofluorophosphate or a combination of both. It is accepted that to be effective, fluoride toothpaste should contain a minimum of 1000 parts per million (ppm) F. In the United Kingdom, the maximum concentration of fluoride that can be sold directly to the public is 1500 ppm F. Fluoride toothpastes containing 2800 ppm F and 5000 ppm F are available on prescription for use by adolescents and adults at particularly high caries risk, on the advice of a dental professional.

Factors that influence the clinical effectiveness of toothpaste in preventing dental caries are summarized in Table 25.1.

The safety of fluoride

Excess consumption of fluoride during the period of tooth formation (Tables 25.2 and 25.3) can result in fluorosis. Steps to avoid exposure in young children are described in Table 25.1.

Acute toxicity can occur if someone is exposed to levels of fluoride in excess of 5 mg F/kg body weight. For a child weighing 10 kg, ingestion of 50 mg F will probably constitute a toxic dose. This equates to 50 g of a 1000 ppm F toothpaste or 33.3 g of a 1500 ppm F toothpaste.

In the event of a suspected acute overdose, if the exposure is < 5 mg/kg body weight, drink large volumes of milk and seek medical advice. If exposure is > 5 mg/kg body weight, refer the individual to hospital for gastric lavage without delay.

Other active ingredients in toothpaste

In addition to fluoride, toothpastes can contain other active ingredients, aimed at improving oral health (Table 25.2).

Table 25.2 Ingredients in toothpaste

Condition against which toothpaste is directed	Active ingredient(s)	Notes
Dental caries	Fluoride	The most common therapeutic agent in toothpastes.
Dental caries	Arginine and calcium salts	Recent studies suggest that addition of arginine and calcium salts to fluoride toothpaste may enhance its anticaries effect, possibly by affecting the pH of the plaque biofilm
Periodontal disease	Antimicrobial agents, e.g. Triclosan	Designed to have antimicrobial effects on periodontopathic organisms
Oral malodour	Antimicrobial agents, e.g. Triclosan	
Calculus	Zinc citrate, pyrophosphate	Toothpastes containing these ingredients have been shown to slow down the accumulation of supra-gingival calculus
Erosion	Fluoride	High-dose fluoride toothpaste may be useful in combating dental erosion
Dentine sensitivity	Potassium chloride, arginine, strontium chloride	Can be helpful when dentine sensitivity is acute
Tooth discolouration	Low-dose peroxide, microparticles	Tooth-whitening toothpastes are currently very popular. May have an abrasive or chemical action or both. While they may remove extrinsic staining, they have no effect on intrinsic staining
Other ingredients in toothpaste		
	Abrasive	To provide efficient cleaning. In times past 'smokers' toothpaste' had abrasives that could result in significant tooth-surface loss. However, *in vitro* tests suggest that the abrasives in modern toothpastes are such that it would takes many years to remove 1 mm of tooth structure
	Humectants and binders	These serve to stop the toothpaste drying out and to combine the ingredients
	Detergents and surfactants	The detergents help loosen debris and make the toothpaste foam
	Flavours, preservatives and colouring	

26 Water fluoridation

Table 26.1 Milestones in the history of water fluoridation

Date	Milestone
1915	**Colorado stain and caries risk**. Fredrick McKay, a public health dentist in Colorado, USA, reported a developmental defect affecting the teeth of local residents. This was shown to be due to the presence of excess fluoride in the drinking water. Natural fluoridation occurs due the local geology. Fluoride is absorbed by water flowing over fluoride-rich rocks and soil on its way to the storage reservoir/aquifer. Crucially, McKay also observed that those affected by fluorosis were less likely to experience dental decay.
1933	**Dean and optimal fluoridation**. Another American public health dentist, Trendly Dean, reported that when fluoride was present at the level of one part per million (1 ppm), the prevalence of dental caries was still low, while fluorosis was also mild.
1945	**The first artificial fluoridation study**. Evidence from the observational studies of McKay, Dean and others in the first half of the twentieth century led to the hypothesis that addition of fluoride to the public water supply could act as a caries-preventive measure. The first such study involved three cities in the US state of Michigan. Fluoride was added to the water supply of the town of Grand Rapids (were the water supply was deficient in fluoride). The city of Muskegon (also lacking fluoride) acted as a control, while the town of Aurora, which was naturally fluoridated, acted as a positive control. After 6.5 years, the prevalence of dental caries in Grand Rapids had fallen by 50%, at which time Muskegon also fluoridated its water supply.
1950	The Medical Research Council's UK studies.
1980	**The Strathclyde Fluoridation Case**. This lengthy legal case established that the only impediment to water fluoridation in Scotland at the time was the lack of legal authority to do so on the part of Strathclyde Council. Representations on the idea of 'mass medication' and the adverse health effects of fluoride were rejected by the court.
1985	**The 1985 Water (Fluoridation) Act**. This stated: 'When requested by a health authority, the water supplier *may*, while the application remains in force, increase the fluoride content of the water supplied by them within that area.' The word 'may' in this legislation was a crucial impediment to the implementation of fluoridation schemes in the United Kingdom. Following privatization of the water industry, water companies chose to interpret the legislation as permissive rather than obligatory. Concerns over who would be responsible for indemnity in the event of an accident also hindered the implementation of fluoridation.
2000	**The York Review**. This government-commissioned systematic review examined the clinical effectiveness and safety of water fluoridation. It established that fluoridation did reduce the prevalence of dental caries. The only adverse outcome was an increased prevalence of fluorosis in fluoridated areas. There was no credible evidence that fluoridation had an adverse impact on general health.
2002	**Medical Research Council Review**. This review suggested the need for research on the public's perception of fluorosis; trends on exposure to fluoride in an era of widespread fluoride toothpaste use; and effects of fluoridation on the oral health of adults.
2003	**Water Act 2003 Section 58 (Fluoridation of Water supplies)**. This clarified indemnity issues (the government would be responsible) and removed water companies' veto, saying that they had to fluoridate if asked to by the Strategic Health Authorities. However, Health Authorities were, as a result of this legislation, required to consult with the local population prior to implementation of a new water-fluoridation scheme.
2007	**Australian National Health and Medical Research Council**. This review concluded that 'the existing body of evidence strongly suggests that fluoridation is beneficial for reducing dental caries'.
2015	**Cochrane Review.** Raised doubts about the quality and age of the evidence supporting fluoridation.

*F*luoridation = the adjustment of the level of fluoride in public water supplies with the intention of preventing dental caries.

The addition of fluoride to the public water supply as a means of preventing dental caries has been practised for nearly 70 years. Key milestones in the fluoridation story are highlighted in Table 26.1. The Centers for Disease Control (CDC) in America have described water fluoridation as one of the 10 great public health achievements of the twentieth century.

The global epidemiology of water fluoridation

According to the British Fluoridation Society, worldwide some 337 million people receive artificially fluoridated water. A further 18 million drink water in which fluoride is naturally present at an optimal level to prevent dental caries. Fluoridation is widespread in the United States. Around 208 million Americans receive optimally fluoridated water – about 74% of the population. Of the 50 largest American cities, 47 have optimally fluoridated water. In Canada, population coverage is estimated at 44%. Fluoridation schemes are widespread in South America (Brazil 41%, Chile 65%), and many countries in Asia are extensively fluoridated – Singapore (100%), Hong Kong (100%) and Malaysia (75%). Fluoridation is very much less widespread in Europe. Only Spain (11%), the Republic of Ireland (73%), Serbia (3%) and England (10%) fluoridate their water supplies. The epidemiology of fluoridation in the United Kingdom is discussed in Box 26.1.

Dental Public Health at a Glance, First Edition. Ivor G. Chestnutt.
© 2016 John Wiley & Sons, Ltd. Published 2016 by John Wiley & Sons, Ltd.

The effectiveness of water fluoridation

Three systematic reviews have investigated the clinical effectiveness of water fluoridation. The York Review concluded that the best available evidence suggests that fluoridation of drinking water supplies reduces caries prevalence, both as measured by the proportion of the population who are caries free and by the mean change in the number of decayed missing and filled teeth. Among 5- to 15-year-olds, water fluoridation reduces the number of caries-affected teeth by on average 2.25 teeth per child. This equates to an overall reduction in tooth decay of about 40%. The percentage of children totally free from decay in fluoridated areas is on average 14.6% higher than in comparable non-fluoridated areas. An Australian review stated that water should be fluoridated at a level between 0.6 and 1.1 ppm, depending on climate, to balance the reduction of dental caries and occurrence of dental fluorosis. A 2015 Cochrane review has noted the lack of contemporary evidence for the effects of fluoridation.

Traditionally water fluoridation has been implemented at a concentration of 1 ppm F. In recent times, concerns over fluorosis and fluoride availability from other sources such as toothpastes has led to a reduction to 0.5–0.8 ppm F in countries where fluoridation is practised.

The ethics of water fluoridation

The ethical aspects of water fluoridation were investigated by the Nuffield Council on Bioethics. It concluded that the argument of 'a coercive intervention' should not be accepted when the addition of a substance to the public water supply brought a health benefit. The acceptability of any public health policy involving the water supply should be considered in relation to:
• the balance of risks and benefits
• the potential for alternatives that rank lower on the intervention ladder to achieve the same outcome
• the role of consent where there are potential harms.
It was concluded that the most appropriate way of deciding whether to fluoridate the water supply was to rely on local democratic decision-making procedures.

Factors necessary for implementation of water fluoridation schemes

For fluoridation to be feasible, a public water supply should be present at a sufficient scale to make the scheme economically viable. Fluoride is added to the water under carefully controlled conditions at the water-treatment works. The population served by these works needs to be sufficiently large and the prevalence of caries needs to be sufficiently high to make a fluoridation scheme economically viable. Areas where the population is served by multiple small reservoirs or wells and bore holes (e.g. rural areas) are not suitable for fluoridation. In addition to these practical considerations, political will and the necessary finance have to be present for fluoridation to be possible.

Objections to water fluoridation

There is a small but vocal minority of individuals who are vehemently opposed to water fluoridation. Over the years a large number of diseases, including bone fracture and various cancers, have been cited as resulting from the presence of fluoride in the public

---

Box 26.1 Water fluoridation in the UK

In the United Kingdom, artificial fluoridation schemes operate only in England. The major fluoridation schemes operate in the West Midlands and the North East – these schemes cover 5.8 million people. A further 0.3 million live in areas where fluoride is naturally present in the water supply at a level sufficient to prevent dental caries.

Following devolution in 1999, the position of the constituent countries of the United Kingdom varied with respect to fluoridation. In England, the Department of Health has since 1998 actively pursued the implementation of new fluoridation schemes in areas of high caries prevalence, but to date without success. In Scotland, failed attempts to introduce fluoridation in the 1980s and early 1990s led to the pursuit of alternative community fluoridation programmes in the guise of the 'Childsmile' programme. The Welsh government accepts the benefits of water fluoridation, but has no plans to implement it and, like Scotland, has opted for a school-based supervised tooth-brushing programme, 'Designed to Smile'.

The reduction in caries prevalence observed in the United Kingdom in recent decades means that fluoridation should be targeted to areas where caries prevalence remains high. This position is supported by the British Dental Association.

---

water supply. Possible adverse effects of fluoridation have been examined in systematic reviews. A meta-regression conducted as part of the York Review found no association between bone fractures and fluoridation. Similarly, no association was demonstrable between fluoridation and the incidence or mortality from any form of cancer.

Other objections raised by anti-fluoridationists include: fluoridation is a form of mass medication; fluoridation is a means of disposing of waste fluoride products from industry; most of the water that has been fluoridated is never ingested by humans; fluoridated water poses a danger to patients undergoing kidney dialysis; and infusion of fluoride while bathing poses a health risk.

Dental fluorosis and fluoridation

While no adverse effects of fluoridation on general health have been established, it is accepted that the prevalence of dental fluorosis is increased in areas were the water supply is fluoridated. This is hardly surprising, given how the caries-preventive effect of fluoride was first discovered (Table 26.1). The degree to which this increase in fluorosis is a problem is a matter of debate.

The economics of water fluoridation

The economics of water fluoridation is related to the caries prevalence and size of the population to be served. The greater the caries prevalence and the larger the number of people served, the more effective the scheme becomes. The costs arise from the capital expenditure required to install the machinery necessary to add and monitor the fluoride. There are then the annual running costs. According to the British Fluoridation Society, a consultation by the South Central Strategic Health Authority in 2008–09 estimated the costs of installing the plant at £471,000, with annual running costs of £59,000. This scheme was designed to serve a population of 195 000 – equating to annual running costs of about 30p per head once the scheme was set up.

The Centers for Disease Control suggest that in the United States, for every $1 spent on water fluoridation, $38 is saved on dental treatment costs.

27 Community fluoride schemes and fissure-sealant programmes

Table 27.1 Community fluoride schemes – evidence, advantages and disadvantages

School-based supervised tooth brushing

Evidence	Advantages	Disadvantages
Randomized controlled trials have shown school tooth brushing to be effective Recommended by NICE oral health improvement guidelines	• Encourages tooth brushing in at-risk children • Socializes tooth brushing • Can achieve very high participation rates due to peer pressure among children in schools	• Expensive • Requires excellent cooperation with schools and education staff • Labour intensive

Fluoride varnish schemes

Evidence	Advantages	Disadvantages
Good evidence for the effectiveness of fluoride varnish when used on an individual basis in clinic Evidence of benefits when used in a population-based programme are still being determined	• Can be targeted at high-risk children • Do not require clinics to deliver • Can be delivered by trained dental nurses	• Require access to at-risk children • Do not necessarily encourage the uptake of tooth brushing in non-tooth-brushers

Fluoride table and drop distribution schemes

Evidence	Advantages	Disadvantages
Limited evidence of effectiveness at current rates of caries prevalence	• None	• Least likely to be taken up by parents of children at greatest risk • Overenthusiastic use risks overdose and fluorosis • Do not socialize routine oral hygiene behaviours – medicalize dental caries • Rely on an outdated understanding of anticaries effects of fluoride

Fluoride mouth-rinsing programmes

Evidence	Advantages	Disadvantages
Evidence of effectiveness comes mainly from the USA, where school mouth-rinse programmes have operated for many years. Suggests more effective in areas of high caries prevalence.	• Can be carried out with relatively limited disruption to school activities • Can be targeted at high-risk children	• Cannot be used in children aged < 8 years

Fluoride in milk

Evidence	Advantages	Disadvantages
Evidence of effectiveness is outdated or from countries where caries prevalence is much greater than is currently the case in the UK	• None over alternatives such as fluoride varnish schemes or supervised school tooth brushing	• Relies on a school milk programme being present • Unclear whether fluoride is present at a sufficient concentration to have a beneficial effect – may simply add to background levels of fluoride without beneficial therapeutic effect

Fluoridated salt

Evidence	Advantages	Disadvantages
Evidence is old and from a time when the caries prevalence was much higher than that currently prevailing	• None – an outdated concept that has no relevance to current dental public health practice	• General public health messages are to reduce salt intake • Cannot easily be targeted to at-risk groups • Issue of whether the fluoride is present at a sufficient concentration intraorally

Dental Public Health at a Glance, First Edition. Ivor G. Chestnutt.
© 2016 John Wiley & Sons, Ltd. Published 2016 by John Wiley & Sons, Ltd.

In the absence of water fluoridation, alternative means of increasing the contact of teeth with fluoride have been devised. Each has advantages and disadvantages (Table 27.1).

National Institute for Health and Care Excellence (NICE) guidelines on oral health improvement

The Health and Social Care Act (2012) transferred responsibility for oral health improvement programmes in England from the National Health Service to local authorities. NICE has issued guidance to local authorities on how to improve oral health in at-risk groups. This guidance supplements and is meant to be used in conjunction with *Delivering Better Oral Health (DBOH) – An Evidence-Based Toolkit for Prevention*, a joint publication by the Department of Health and the British Association for the Study of Community Dentistry. DBOH deals mainly with improving oral health at an individual level, while the NICE guidance deals with populations or high-risk groups within the general population (Chapter 23).

School-based supervised tooth brushing

Supervised tooth brushing in schools has been used as an alternative to water fluoridation in some countries. The 'Childsmile' programme in Scotland (www.child-smile.org.uk) takes a whole-population approach, while the 'Designed to Smile' programme in Wales (www.designedtosmile.co.uk) takes a targeted-population approach, whereby the programme is directed at those deemed at greatest risk.

Fluoride varnish programmes

Fluoride varnish programmes have been introduced in areas of high dental need. Systematic reviews have shown that application of fluoride varnish 2–4 times per year has a caries-preventive effect. NICE guidelines recommend this approach for children in nursery school aged 3 and over in areas of high caries prevalence. The most commonly used fluoride varnish contains fluoride at a concentration of 22 600 ppm F.

Fluoride tablet and drop distribution schemes

In the 1970s and 1980s, fluoride tablet and drop distribution schemes were popular in the United Kingdom. This was at a time when the systemic effect of fluoride (incorporation of fluoride into the tooth enamel during mineralization) was thought to be the mechanism whereby fluoride increased resistance to bacterial acids. A changed understanding of how fluoride exerts its caries-protective effects (topical) plus poor compliance by the parents of those children at greatest risk have led to the abandonment of these schemes. There may be a role for fluoride tablets and drops on an individual basis prescribed by dental professionals, although they are currently more likely to use a fluoride varnish than to prescribe fluoride tablets and drops.

Fluoride mouth-rinsing programmes

Weekly mouth-rinsing programmes with a 0.2% NaF (sodium fluoride) solution were once very common in the United States. There are currently no school-based mouth-rinsing programmes in the United Kingdom and it is not recommended as a community fluoride scheme. Daily mouth rinsing on an individual basis with a fluoride rinse containing 0.05% NaF is recommended for individuals at high risk of caries as a supplement to twice-daily tooth brushing. Mouthwashes are not recommended for children aged under 8 years. To maximize intraoral fluoride concentration, mouthwashes should be used at a different time of the day from tooth brushing.

Fluoride in milk

For many years, school milk has been seen as a potential means of increasing the availability of fluoride to children and some limited milk-fluoridation schemes still operate in the northwest of England. Elsewhere in the world they are more common and large schemes have been implemented in Russia, Chile and Thailand. Much of the work to continue milk fluoridation has been facilitated by the Borrow Foundation, a charity that has as its aim improving oral health through the greater use of fluorides, particularly via milk and milk products. Fluoridated milk is not formally recommended in current NICE guidelines.

Fluoridated salt

The addition of fluoride to salt began in some European countries, mainly Switzerland and France, in the mid-twentieth century and claims for a caries-protective effect have been made. This concept followed the addition of iodine to salt as a measure to combat goitre. Only 10% of salt intake is added by individuals to their food – the vast majority of salt is added to food during the manufacturing process. Attempts have been made to persuade bakers to use fluoridated salt in bread making. However, given the general health message about reducing the overall intake of salt to protect cardiovascular health, fluoridated salt is no longer regarded as a realistic oral health protection measure in the United Kingdom.

Fluoride gels and foams

Fluoride gels and foams applied in individual trays were used in the past. However, these were only ever suitable for use on an individual patient basis in a dental clinic. They have largely been superseded by fluoride varnish.

Fissure-sealant programmes

In addition to community fluoride programmes, school-based fissure-sealant programmes have been promoted. These aim specifically to deal with dental caries occurring on the occlusal surface of first permanent molar teeth. The majority (80%) of tooth decay in teenagers is to be found on the occlusal surfaces of first permanent molars.

Fissure sealants are Bis-GMA (bisphenol A-glycidyl methacrylate) based materials that are attached to the pit and fissure surface of the teeth using acid-etch technology. They work by providing a physical barrier to the accumulation of a cariogenic plaque biofilm in the depths of the crevices, thereby reducing caries susceptibility. For maximal effectiveness they should be applied shortly after the teeth erupt (when they are particularly caries susceptible) and should be maintained and replaced if they are lost or become defective.

A recent systematic review has shown that concerns about decay progression under sealants are unfounded. This means that unless there is clear evidence that the caries process has progressed into the dentine, occlusal surfaces can be sealed.

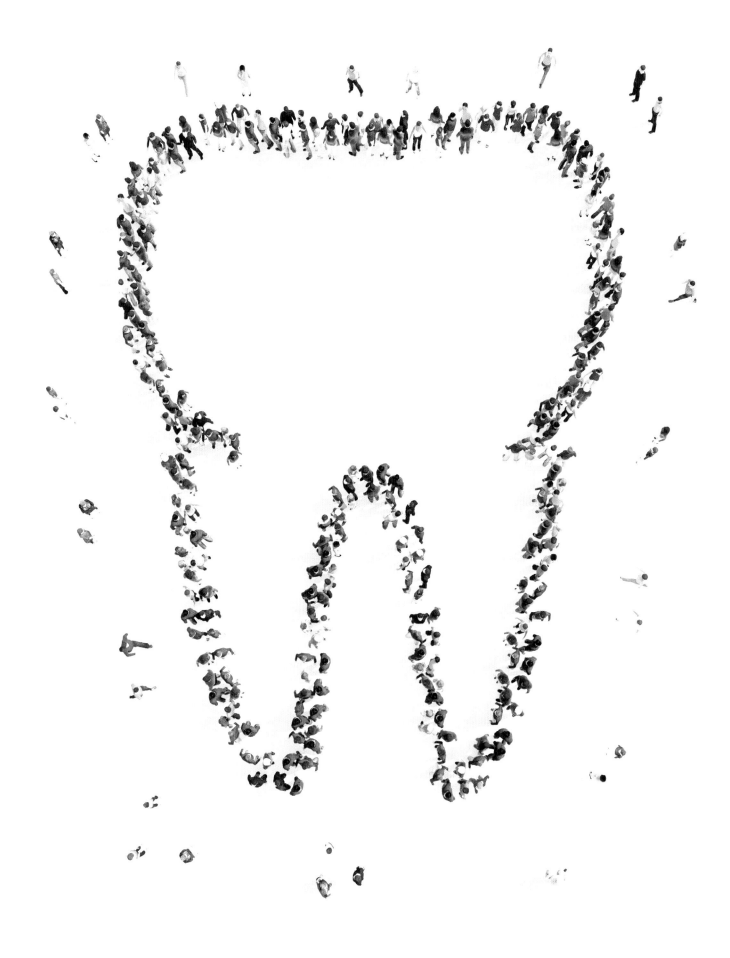

Diet and oral health

Chapters

28 Diet and oral health

Figure 28.1a Effect of diet on oral health

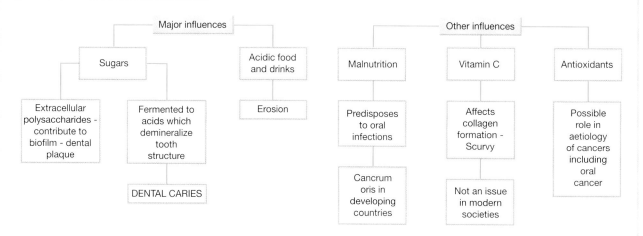

Figure 28.1b Effect of oral health on diet

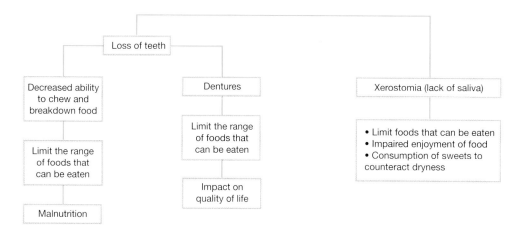

Figure 28.2 Effect of repeated sugar intake on the pH of the oral biofilm

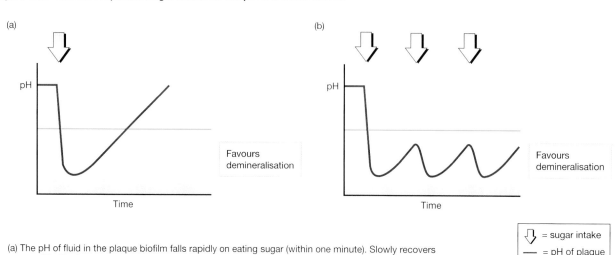

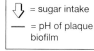

= sugar intake

= pH of plaque biofilm

(a) The pH of fluid in the plaque biofilm falls rapidly on eating sugar (within one minute). Slowly recovers over 20–40 minutes as pH rises due to buffering and washing effect of saliva, sugar used up.
(b) Repeated intakes of sugar mean that pH remains for prolonged period below the point which favours demineralisation.

Dental Public Health at a Glance, First Edition. Ivor G. Chestnutt.
© 2016 John Wiley & Sons, Ltd. Published 2016 by John Wiley & Sons, Ltd.

Diet and health

A good diet and adequate nutrition are essential for health. Poor diet is a key risk factor for many chronic diseases, including cardiovascular disease, diabetes, cancers, osteoporosis, gastrointestinal disorders and dental caries. The sedentary lifestyle of modern populations coupled with the ease of access to energy-rich food and drink has led to an increasing proportion of the population being overweight or obese. The relationship between diet and oral health works in two ways. Diet is an important predisposing risk factor for oral disease, most notably dental caries. Conversely, oral health can have an impact on diet and nutrition (Figures 28.1a and 28.1b).

A common risk factor approach to health improvement means that messages about reducing the amount and frequency of sugar consumption that relate to oral health relate also to general health.

Diet and dental caries

Evidence that sugar in the diet is responsible for dental caries comes from different types of study.
- **Animal studies:** Many of the early investigations into the effect of sugar on dental caries involved the use of animals (most commonly rats).
- **In-situ appliance experiments:** In these experiments enamel slabs are mounted on intraoral appliances (i.e. part dentures that clip over teeth) and are worn by volunteers (often dental students!). Sugar solutions of varying type and concentration are applied to the slabs *ex vivo* and the appliance is inserted and worn for varying periods. The plaque biofilm is then 'fed' with sugar. The degree of de/remineralization of the enamel slab can be detected by removal of the slab from the appliance and use of microradiography.
- **Human plaque pH studies:** An in-dwelling pH electrode can be used to measure plaque pH in real time, as acids are produced by fermentation following the ingestion of a sugar-containing solution or foodstuff. This type of study can be used to demonstrate the effect of frequency of sugar intake. Repeated exposure to sugar replenishes the sugar supply to the bacteria in the plaque biofilm. As a result, buffers in saliva and the washing effect of saliva are negated, and the pH at the tooth surface favours the net loss of calcium and phosphate ions (demineralization) for as long as the repeated sugar consumption continues (Figure 28.2).
- **Observational studies:** Many studies on the role of sugar and dental caries take the form of observational studies, where the relationship is examined at (cross-sectional) or over (longitudinal) a period of time.
- **Cross-sectional studies**
  - *Country by country analysis:* A significant correlation between sugar consumption per capita and caries prevalence has been shown on a country-by-country basis. Caries levels are low when total sugar consumption is less than 10 kg/person/year, but increase rapidly when sugar consumption rises above 15 kg/person/year. This is a crude measure and takes no account of the variation of sugar consumption by individuals, and it also does not account for the frequency of sugar consumption.
  - *Communities with special diets:* The prevalence of dental caries has been examined in communities with special diets that either consume excess sugar or have a sugar-restricted diet. Confectionery workers who were at liberty to consume their products have been shown to be at greater risk for dental caries, while hereditary fructose intolerance, a developmental metabolic defect that requires a diet low in sugar, has a low caries prevalence.
- **Longitudinal studies and serial cross-sectional before-and-after studies:** Past studies have shown changes in caries prevalence following changes in the availability of sugar. Wartime studies demonstrate that the prevalence of dental caries fell during the Second World War when sugar became scarce, and rose again following the increased availability of sugar when hostilities ended. Further evidence comes from remote communities whose traditional diet was low in sugar, which experienced increased caries levels when introduced to sugar-rich diets. One of the most often-quoted examples is the remote Atlantic island of Tristan da Cunha, where the oral health of the population deteriorated following the establishment of an American defence base and the resultant increased availability of sugar.
- **Intervention studies:** Manipulation of diet in an experimental setting is difficult, but there are a few often-quoted studies that have attempted this relating to oral health. The famous Vipeholm study conducted in a mental hospital in Sweden in the 1950s fed patients in different wards sugar in various formats. Many criticisms can be made of that study from an experimental and particularly ethical perspective. However, data from that study have been used to demonstrate the detrimental effects of sugar when consumed frequently and in sticky retentive forms. Another example is the Turku studies in Finland, which investigated the effects of xylitol on caries de- and remineralization.

The quality of the evidence that sugar causes dental caries

The evidence that sugar causes dental caries is incontrovertible. However, the majority of the studies referred to were conducted in the era before fluoride was widely available in communities, either in the public water supply or in toothpaste.

Breastfeeding and dental caries

Wherever possible, new mothers should be encouraged to breastfeed – the benefits to children of breastfeeding exceed those of bottle feeding. However, there have been some reports of dental caries associated with abnormal patterns of breastfeeding, where the child is allowed to feed 'ad libitum'; that is, at will and throughout the night.

Diet and dental erosion

A diet with a high acidic content can cause erosion of the teeth. This is most commonly seen in individuals who consume large quantities of carbonated beverages, particularly those who consume acidic drinks at frequent intervals through the day. Erosion can also be seen in people who eat excessive quantities of acidic fruits such as citrus fruits and green apples.

Diet and periodontal disease

Periodontal disease in not influenced by diet to any extent. Vitamin C deficiency (scurvy) affects collagen formation, but this condition is unlikely to be encountered in dental practice.

Public health aspects of dietary modification

Figure 29.1 Forest plot of the relationship between obesity and dental caries. Source: *Hayden et al. 2013. Reproduced with permission from John Wiley & Sons.*

Group by	Study name	Statistics for each study				Std diff in means and 95% CI
Dentition type		Std diff in means	Lower limit	Upper limit	P-value	
Permanent	Alm et al., 2008	0.474	−0.062	1.010	0.083	
Permanent	Gerdin et al., 2008	0.096	0.017	0.175	0.017	
Permanent	Granville-Garcia et al., 2008	−0.027	−0.282	0.228	0.836	
Permanent	Narksawat et al. 2009	−0.530	−0.809	−0.252	0.000	
Permanent	Sadeghi and Alizadch, 2007 (permanent teeth)	0.394	0.176	0.612	0.000	
Permanent	Sharma and Hedge, 2009	0.370	0.078	0.661	0.013	
Permanent	Tramini et al., 2009	0.095	−0.259	0.450	0.599	
Permanent	Willerhausen et al., 2007 (permanent teeth)	0.239	0.053	0.425	0.012	
Permanent		0.124	−0.053	0.301	0.170	
Primary	Chenetal, 1998	0.034	−0.080	0.148	0.562	
Primary	Kopycka-Kedzierawski et al., 2008 (primary teeth)	−0.123	−0.386	0.140	0.360	
Primary	Macek and Mitola, 2008	0.140	−0.038	0.319	0.124	
Primary	Oliveira et al., 2008	−0.282	−0.563	0.000	0.050	
Primary	Sadeghi and Alizadch, 2007 (primary teeth)	0.227	0.010	0.445	0.040	
Primary	Sheller et al., 2009	0.094	−0.353	0.541	0.681	
Primary	Vazquez-Nava et al., 2009	0.362	0.179	0.544	0.000	
Primary	Willerhausen et al., 2007 (primary teeth)	0.159	−0.027	0.345	0.093	
Primary		0.093	−0.033	0.220	0.149	
Overall		0.104	0.001	0.206	0.049	

−1.00 −0.50 0.00 0.50 1.00
Favours non-caries Favours caries

Meta analysis

A non-significant relationship is observed between obesity and dental caries in the permanent dentition (p = 0.17) and in the primary dentition (p = 0.149). A marginally significant relationship is observed when both primary and permanent dentition are combined (p = 0.049)

Table 29.1 Definitions of overweight and obesity

Children < 5 years old

Overweight	Weight for height >±2 standard deviations (SD) of the WHO Child Growth Standards median

School-aged children and adolescents (5–19 years old)

Overweight	Body Mass Index (BMI) for age >+1 SD of the WHO growth reference for school-aged children and adolescents (equivalent to BMI 25 kg/m² at 19 years)
Obese	>±2 standard deviations of the WHO growth reference for school-aged children and adolescents (equivalent to BMI 30 kg/m² at 19 years)

Adults (> 20 years)

Overweight	BMI > 25 kg/m²
Obese	BMI > 30 kg/m²

Data source: *WHO*

$$BMI = \frac{mass\ (kg)}{height\ (m)^2}$$

Box 29.1 Recommended sugars intake

- WHO recommends a reduced intake of free sugars throughout the lifecourse (strong recommendation).
- In both adults and children, WHO recommends reducing the intake of free sugars to less than 10% of total energy intake (strong recommendation).
- WHO suggests a further reduction of the intake of free sugars to below 5% of total energy intake (conditional recommendation).

Source: *WHO 2015. Reproduced with permission from World Health Organization.*

Box 29.2 Suggested actions to reduce obesity

- Multisectoral population-based policies to influence production, marketing and consumption of healthy foods.
- Fiscal policies to increase the availability and consumption of healthy food and reduce consumption of unhealthy food.
- Promotion of breastfeeding.
- Policies and actions to reduce physical inactivity.
- Educational and social marketing campaigns focused on appropriate diet and increasing physical activity.
- Policies to reduce direct marketing and advertising of foods high in sugar and fat to children.
- Introduction of measures to create healthy eating environments.

Source: *WHO 2015. Reproduced with permission from World Health Organization.*

Free sugars

Free sugars are defined by the World Health Organization (WHO) as:

Monosaccharides and disaccharides added to foods and beverages by the manufacturer, cook or consumer, and sugars naturally present in honey, syrups, fruit juices and juice concentrates.

This includes sucrose and its constituent parts fructose and glucose. Free sugars contribute to the energy density of foods. The ready availability of such foods and the consumption of them, especially sugar-sweetened beverages, can easily lead to an excess of energy intake over energy expenditure.

Recommended sugar intake

The WHO has issued guidance on the intake of sugar. Energy intake from free sugars should comprise less than 10% of energy intake and ideally would be less than 5% of total energy intake (Box 29.1).

Obesity

One of the greatest challenges to the public's health is the ever-increasing proportion of the population who are either overweight or obese. According to the WHO, worldwide obesity has more than doubled since 1980 and in 2014, 11% of men and 15% of women aged 18 years and older were obese. Globally, an estimated 42 million children under the age of 5 years were overweight in 2013.

According to Public Health England, in 2013, 26% of English men and 23.8% of women were obese. It is estimated that by 2050, 60% of men, 50% of women and 25% of children will be obese. Obesity has been described as the new smoking and some authorities have suggested that the challenges posed by sugar in the twenty-first century equate to those posed by tobacco in the twentieth century.

Definitions of overweight and obesity are shown in Table 29.1. Suggested actions to tackle obesity are shown in Box 29.2.

Obesity and dental caries

Obesity and dental caries have in common a major dietary component in their aetiology, and in particular the consumption of sweetened beverages. However, epidemiological studies have been somewhat equivocal in demonstrating a consistent relationship between obesity and caries, some studies showing a significant association while others fail to demonstrate such a relationship. A recent systematic review (Hayden et al. 2012) found a marginally significant association across all dentition types, but not separately for primary and permanent teeth (Figure 29.1). A further analysis by those authors using standardized measures of obesity demonstrated a more significant relationship between obesity and caries in the permanent teeth.

These findings reflect the multifactorial aetiology of both obesity and dental caries. The assumption that children who eat more are more likely to experience decay is possibly mistaken. Underweight children may well have a food intake that comprises frequent sugar-rich drinks and confectionery.

Actions to reduce sugar intake

- **Fruit tuck shops:** Many schools have banned 'tuck shops' that sell sweets and sugar-rich drinks and replaced them with shops that sell only fruit.
- **Water in schools:** In a similar vein, many schools now allow children to have a bottle of water at their desk. Many insist on transparent bottles so that the contents can be clearly seen. Not only do water-in-school schemes encourage the consumption of a tooth-friendly drink (i.e. water), the children are adequately hydrated.
- **Vending machines:** A ban on vending machines selling sweetened drinks has been implemented in hospitals and schools in Wales. This is a good practical example of creating a healthier environment as set out in the Ottawa Charter (Chapter 20).
- **Sweet-free checkouts:** A long-standing campaign has been conducted to persuade the major supermarkets to remove sweets and confectionery from check-outs, where placed at child's eye level they are positioned to facilitate maximum '**pester power**' at the end of a shopping trip. This campaign has met with partial success in that most supermarkets now offer at least some sweet-free check-outs.
- **Advertising directed at children:** Previous research has demonstrated that a significantly greater proportion of television advertisements during children's television time in late afternoon was for foods and drinks than was the case at prime time during the evening. Advertisements for sugar-rich cereals were particularly common. Recent changes to advertising regulations have placed greater restrictions on how sugar-rich products are targeted at children.

Sugar substitutes

Food manufacturers have explored alternatives to sucrose and fructose as sweetening agents in 'diet' or 'light' drinks, including saccharine, aspartame and xylitol. As these agents are not broken down by oral bacteria, such drinks are not cariogenic. However, as the carbonation process means that 'diet' drinks inherently have a very low pH, frequent consumption poses a risk of dental erosion.

Confectionery that uses sugar substitutes as sweetening agents is manufactured and sold using the 'tooth-friendly' logo. Sugar alcohols such as xylitol are used here. However, the side effects of xylitol consumption limit their use, particularly in young children in whom excess intake can lead to diarrhoea.

The greatest issue yet to be overcome by food scientists is the lack of heat resistance of current sugar substitutes. This limits their use in cooked and baked foods.

Sugar tax

Growing awareness of the obesity epidemic has led in some quarters to a call for a tax to be placed on sugared food. Increasing taxation has been a successful tool in reducing tobacco consumption. However, while tobacco is not a prerequisite for life, people do need to eat. The best way of taxing foodstuffs to encourage people to eat more healthily has still to be established.

Sugar industry

Clearly, those involved in the production and marketing of sugar-containing products are resistant to attempts to constrain the market in sugars, and the sugar industry has opposed WHO guidelines on the intake of sugars. One interesting recent development is the publication of a paper that reviewed a historical archive of papers at the National Institute of Dental Research, the body responsible for setting the dental research agenda in the United States. This analysis by Kearns et al., published in 2015, suggests that the US 1971 National Caries Programme was deflected by the sugar industry to public health interventions that would reduce the harms of sugar consumption rather than restricting intake. Kearns and colleagues claim that research that could have been harmful to sugar industry interests was omitted from the national research programme.

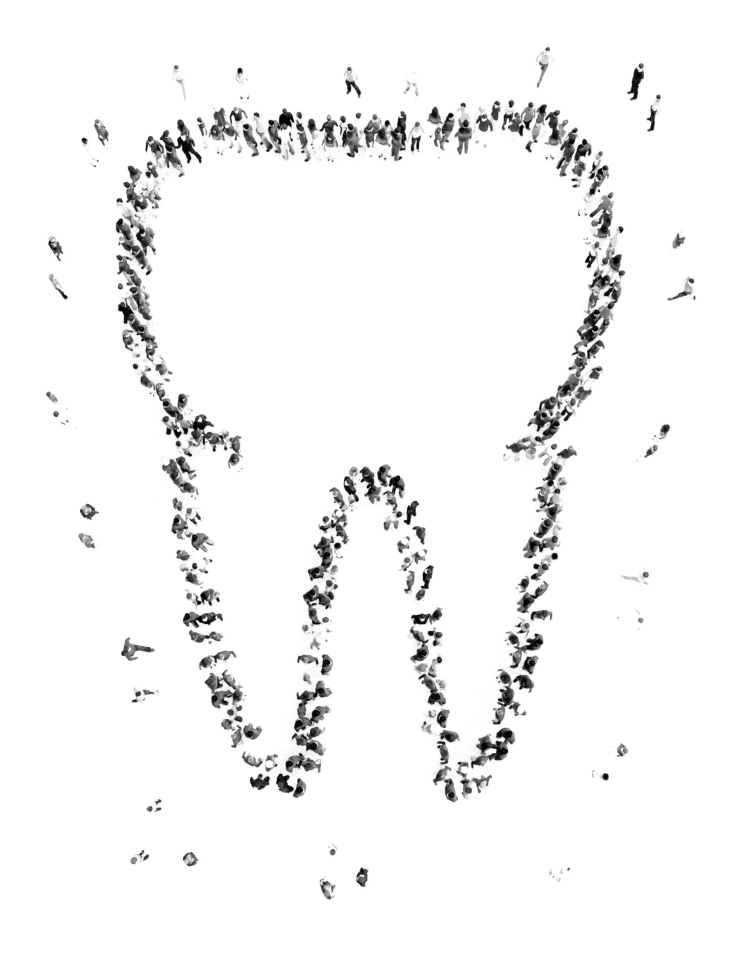

Smoking and oral health

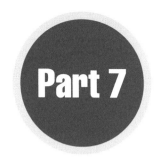

Chapters

30 Smoking and oral health

Figure 30.1 Stages of the worldwide tobacco epidemic. Source: *Edwards 2004. Reproduced with permission from BJM Publishing Group.*

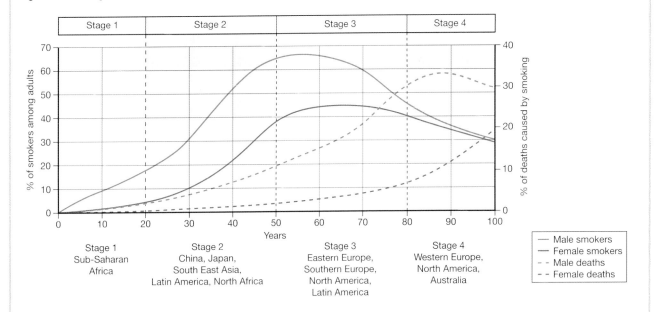

Figure 30.2 Prevalence of smoking in the UK 1974–2011. Source: *Office for National Statistics 2011. Reproduced with permission from Office for National Statistics.*

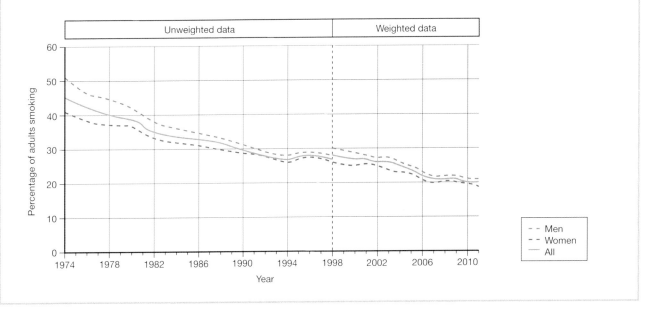

Epidemiology of tobacco use

It is estimated that there are 1 billion smokers worldwide, of whom 80% live in low- and middle-income countries. In the first half of the twentieth century in the United States and Europe, cigarette smoking was extremely common. However, changed attitudes to smoking, increased tobacco control legislation and high-profile legal cases in North America have led tobacco companies to focus their attention on developing countries.

The global pattern of tobacco use is illustrated in Figure 30.1. This shows that while tobacco use has peaked in Western Europe, North America and Australia, in areas such as China, South East Asia and Latin America the peak in tobacco use has still to be reached. The World Health Organization (WHO) reckons that tobacco caused 100 million deaths in the twentieth century and if current trends continue, it may cause 1 billion deaths in the twenty-first century.

The demographics of tobacco smoking in the United Kingdom

Trends in tobacco use in the United Kingdom are shown in Figure 30.2. In 1974 just under half of the adult population smoked tobacco. By 2011 the mean number of smokers had fallen to 1 in 5 adults. Marginally fewer women than men smoke in the United Kingdom. These average data for the total population mask an important fact – the association between smoking and social class. Data from the Welsh Health Survey are shown in Table 30.1. This shows that there is a threefold difference in the prevalence of smoking between managerial and professional classes and the long-term unemployed, where 2 in 5 still smoke.

The prevalence of cigarette smoking varies among different ethnic groups in England (Table 30.2). While 40% of Bangladeshi men smoke, only 2% of Bangladeshi women smoke cigarettes. This contrasts with black Caribbean women resident in England, 24% of whom report smoking. It should be remembered that although cigarette smoking in some ethnic groups may be lower than in the general population, tobacco may be used in alternative formats, such as betel quid (Chapter 31).

Tobacco and general health

According to the WHO, tobacco kills nearly 6 million people each year and it is forecast that unless urgent action is taken, the annual global death toll could rise to more than 8 million by 2030. Tobacco consumption is recognized as the United Kingdom's single greatest cause of preventable illness and early death, with an estimated 102,000 people dying from smoking-related diseases in 2009. The effects of smoking are not confined to those who smoke. **Passive smoking** (breathing tobacco smoke produced by others) can be lethal to non-smokers.

Passive smoking

Non-smokers who live with a smoking partner or who work in an environment where levels of tobacco smoke are high, such as pubs and bars, are at increased risk of developing a smoking-related disease. Recognition of the impact of second-hand tobacco smoke has been instrumental in the introduction of legislation prohibiting smoking in public places. Smoking during pregnancy is likely to have an adverse impact on the health of the foetus.

Tobacco and oral health

Tobacco, whether smoked or used in a smokeless form, has impacts on oral health in many ways (Table 30.3).

Table 30.3 The effect of tobacco use on oral health

Condition	Observations
Hairy tongue	Caused by increased keratinization of the filiform papillae, this is a benign condition that is most commonly seen in smokers. It may assume a brown or black colour due to the presence of chromogenic bacteria.
Halitosis	Probably the most common effect of smoking – can be used as a motivator to encourage young people to quit smoking.
Keratosis	Thickening of the oral mucosa, particularly in areas directly exposed to the thermal trauma of cigarette smoke, results in a white appearance and increased keratin layer on the mucosal surface. Nicotinic stomatitis affecting the palate and buccal mucosa are commonly affected sites.
Leukoplakia	White patches that may be precancerous are more commonly seen in smokers.
Oral cancer	The most serious effect of tobacco use on the oral cavity. Smoking cigarettes increases the risk of oral cancer 2–4 times. Smoking has a synergistic effect when combined with heavy alcohol consumption, which together increase the risk of developing oral cancer 6–15 times.
Periodontal disease	Smoking cigarettes will increase the risk of periodontal attachment loss by 2–5 times. However, periodontal disease in smokers can be masked by the vasoconstrictive effects of nicotine on the gingival tissues, resulting in a lack of bleeding and the obvious redness pathognomonic of gingivitis.
Wound healing	Smokers frequently have an impaired ability to heal – alveolar osteitis (dry socket) is seen more commonly in smokers. Patients who smoke respond less well to both non-surgical and surgical periodontal therapy.
Sinusitis	The irritant effects of cigarette smoke predisposes to sinusitis.
Tooth staining	Smoking, often in combination with poor oral hygiene, is a common cause of external tooth discolouration. Staining can be used as a motivating factor to help discuss smoking cessation in a non-threatening way with patients.

Table 30.1 Prevalence of self-reported cigarette smoking by social class (% current smokers)

Social class	% current smokers
Managerial and professional	14
Intermediate	21
Routine and manual	30
Never worked and long-term unemployed	41

Source: *Welsh Government 2012.*

Table 30.2 Self-reported cigarette smoking status, by minority ethnic group and sex (% current smokers)

Cigarette smoking status	Minority ethnic group							
	Black Caribbean	Black African	Indian	Pakistani	Bangladeshi	Chinese	Irish	General population
Men	25	21	20	29	40	21	30	24
Women	24	10	5	5	2	8	26	23

Source: *Adapted from Health and Social Care Information Centre 2006.*

31 Alternative ways in which tobacco is used and tobacco control

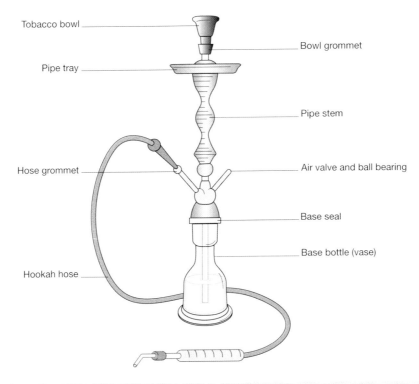

Figure 31.1 Diagrammatic representation of a waterpipe

- Tobacco bowl
- Bowl grommet
- Pipe tray
- Pipe stem
- Air valve and ball bearing
- Hose grommet
- Base seal
- Base bottle (vase)
- Hookah hose

Table 31.1 Summary of the effects of using a waterpipe to smoke tobacco

Using a waterpipe to smoke tobacco poses a serious potential health hazard to smokers and others exposed to the smoke emitted. Using a waterpipe to smoke tobacco is not a safe alternative to cigarette smoking.

A typical one-hour-long waterpipe smoking session involves inhaling 100–200 times the volume of smoke inhaled with a single cigarette.

Even after it has been passed through water, the smoke produced by a waterpipe contains high levels of toxic compounds, including carbon monoxide, heavy metals and cancer-causing chemicals.

Commonly used heat sources that are applied to burn the tobacco, such as wood cinders or charcoal, are likely to increase the health risks, because when such fuels are combusted they produce their own toxicants, including high levels of carbon monoxide, metals and cancer-causing chemicals.

Pregnant women and the foetus are particularly vulnerable when exposed either actively or involuntarily to the waterpipe smoke and toxicants.

Second-hand smoke from waterpipes is a mixture of tobacco smoke in addition to the smoke from the fuel and therefore poses a serious risk for non-smokers.

There is no proof that any device or accessory can make waterpipe smoking safer.

Sharing a waterpipe mouthpiece poses a serious risk of transmission of communicable diseases, including tuberculosis and hepatitis.

Waterpipe tobacco is often sweetened and flavoured, making it very appealing; the sweet smell and taste of the smoke may explain why some people, particularly young people who otherwise would not use tobacco, begin to use waterpipes.

Source: WHO 2005. Reproduced with permission from World Health Organization.

Table 31.2 Recent UK legislation designed to have an effect on tobacco smoking

Legislation	Date introduced	Applicability
Legislation relating to advertisements		
Ban on advertising cigarettes on billboards and in the press and magazines	February 2003	UK wide
Restrictions on advertising at point of sale	December 2004	UK wide
Ban on tobacco displays in shops	June 2011 (large shops) October 2013 (smaller premises)	England
Legislation prohibiting smoking		
Ban on smoking in enclosed work and other public spaces	March 2006 April 2007	Scotland England and Wales
Restriction on sales		
Minimum age at which tobacco can be legally purchased raised from 16 years to 18 years	October 2007	UK wide
Legislation relating to cigarette packaging		
Pictorial warnings on the back of cigarette packets made compulsory	October 2008	UK wide
Plain packaging	Legislation passed by UK parliament March 2015	UK wide

Alternative ways in which tobacco is used

Tobacco is most commonly smoked in the form of cigarettes, either manufactured or as 'roll-ups'. Smoking cigars or a pipe is a less frequent form of consumption. However, it is common in many ethnic groups for tobacco to be used in other ways, all of which are prejudicial to oral health.

Bidis

Bidis are small, hand-rolled cigarettes typically smoked in India and other South East Asian countries. They produce three times more carbon monoxide and five times more tar than regular cigarettes.

Shisha, hookas, waterpipes

Shisha, tobacco cured with flavourings and smoked from **waterpipes** (also known as hookas or hubble-bubbles), is used by an estimated 100 million people worldwide. Originating in Middle Eastern countries, it is becoming increasingly common in Europe and North America. The moistened tobacco is placed in a bowl over hot coals and the smoke drawn by a pipe through water (Figure 31.1). Use of tobacco in this format poses risks to general and oral health (Table 31.1).

Betel quid

Betel quid is a combination of betel leaf, areca nut and slaked lime. With or without tobacco, it is widely used in Asia and the Pacific region. It is also used by people resident in the United Kingdom whose origins are in Asia. Placed in the buccal sulcus, the quid has a mildly stimulant effect. Use predisposes to the development of precancerous conditions: leukoplakia, erythroplakia and oral submucous fibrosis (OSF). OSF is common in the Indian subcontinent and presents as a thickening of the oral soft tissues, which limits opening of the mouth.

Gutkha

Gutkha is a smokeless tobacco mixture that is sweetened and spiced. It is sold in foil packets and the highly coloured packaging makes it attractive to children and young people.

Tobacco and recreational drugs

Cannabis (marijuana) is commonly smoked in combination with tobacco. Smokers of 'weed' commonly present with the intraoral signs common in those who smoke conventional cigarettes.

Dipping tobacco (moist snuff)

This mode of tobacco use originates in Scandinavia. A bolus of tobacco is placed in the buccal sulcus and the nicotine is absorbed via the oral tissues. It is sold either loose in tins or in bags that resemble tea-bags. Its use predisposes the individual to oral cancer. Made popular by American baseball stars, dipping tobacco still poses a problem among US teenagers.

Approaches to tobacco control

Approaches to controlling tobacco can be divided into:
- Control measures aimed at a population level (upstream).
- Control measures aimed at helping individuals stop smoking (downstream).

Population-level tobacco control measures

Health departments in the United Kingdom have introduced a range of tobacco control measures (Table 31.2). The ban on smoking in enclosed work and public spaces is one of the most significant public health measures to have been implemented in recent decades.

Bans on tobacco advertising, promotion and sponsorship can reduce tobacco consumption. Tobacco taxes are one of the most cost-effective ways of reducing tobacco use, especially among young people and the poor. The World Health Organization suggests that a tax increase that raises the price of tobacco by 10% decreases tobacco consumption by about 4% in high-income countries and by up to 8% in low- and middle-income countries. Taxation has over the years been a key weapon against tobacco use in the United Kingdom. However, this means of control is undermined by the ready availability of smuggled, contraband and fake tobacco brands on the black market. In 2010 the UK Border Agency seized 550 million cigarettes that were being imported illegally.

Stopping smoking

Given the impact of tobacco on health, stopping people taking up smoking or helping them cease the habit if they already use tobacco is one of the great challenges facing public health. One half of all smokers will die directly as a result of their habit. In surveys, around 7 in 10 smokers report that they would like to give up smoking, and just under 4 in 10 smokers have tried to do so in the past 12 months. Five out of six smokers claim that they would not start smoking had they the choice to make again.

Nicotine, a psychoactive substance that acts on receptors in the brain, is highly addictive. Overcoming dependence on nicotine is a key element in giving up smoking. Nicotine withdrawal symptoms can include irritability, anxiety, difficulty concentrating and increased appetite. Stopping smoking is difficult and those who successfully quit often report several failed attempts before finally kicking the habit.

The benefits of stopping smoking

Smoking cessation:
- Lowers the risk of lung and other types of cancer.
- Reduces the risk of coronary heart disease, stroke and peripheral vascular disease. Coronary heart disease risk is substantially reduced within one to two years of quitting.
- Reduces respiratory symptoms such as coughing, wheezing and shortness of breath and also reduces the risk of developing chronic obstructive pulmonary disease.
- Reduces staining of the teeth and halitosis.
- Increases the chances of a successful outcome following the placement of dental implants or periodontal surgery.

As described in Chapter 32, members of the dental team have an important role to play in helping smokers give up.

32 Smoking cessation

Figure 32.1 The Stages of Change Model as applied to smoking cessation in a dental setting. Source: *Adapted from Prochaska and DiClemente 1982.*

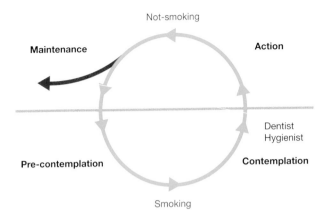

Table 32.1 NHS smoking-cessation websites and helplines

Country	Programme	Website	Helpline
England	NHS Choices Smokefree	www.smokefree.nhs.uk	0800 022 4332
Wales	Stop Smoking Wales	www.stopsmokingwales.com	0800 085 2219
Scotland	Can Stop Smoking	www.canstopsmoking.com	0800 84 84 84
Northern Ireland	NHS Stop Smoking Line		0800 85 85 85

Table 32.2 The four As of tobacco cessation

Task	Action
Ask	Ask all patients about their smoking status.
Advise	Advise on the impact of smoking on oral health and on the adverse effect on the outcomes of dental treatment (e.g. dry sockets, increased implant failures)
Assist	Assist those who express an interest in stopping smoking to access suitable professional help (e.g. by referral to the local smoking-cessation service)
Arrange	At a follow-up appointment ask about progress with cessation and offer encouragement

Individual smoking cessation – the process of stopping smoking

A number of behaviour change theories have been applied to helping individuals stop smoking. One of the most popular is the Stages of Change or Trans-theoretical Model of Change proposed by American psychologists Prochasksa and DiClemente. This model suggests that people move through a series of motivational stages before they succeed in stopping smoking (Figure 32.1). The majority of smokers are at any one time in a **precontemplation stage** (not thinking about quitting). A minority of smokers are at any one time thinking about giving up – the **contemplation stage**. Some will then take action and stop smoking – the **action stage**. Some manage to stay stopped and enter the **maintenance stage** (stopped smoking for more than six months). However, many will fail and relapse before going on to try a further quit attempt.

While some smokers manage to stay stopped after the first attempt, many will go around the quit and relapse circle a number of times before finally managing to stay stopped. In some ways the process can be viewed as learning and practising. Many smoking-cessation programmes aim to identify the stage that a smoker is in at a given time and attempt to tailor cessation information appropriately.

A recent Cochrane review of stage-based interventions for smoking cessation concluded that approaches based on stages of change were neither more nor less effective than interventions that were not based on such an approach.

What helps smokers quit?

While the majority of smokers give up without resort to evidence-based cessation therapies, the evidence base suggests that there are two important components that either alone or in combination will increase the chances of a smoker successfully quitting:
- Advice and counselling
- Medication

Advice and counselling

Brief advice from a healthcare professional will increase the chances of stopping smoking. Counselling either in person, individually or in groups, or via telephone helplines is successful in increasing cessation rates. Interactive websites also provide helpful information and assistance to those who are attempting to stop smoking (Table 32.1).

Medication

Continuance of smoking is heavily influenced by dependence on nicotine. The provision of **nicotine-replacement therapy (NRT)** significantly increases the chances of a successful quit attempt. NRT is available in a range of delivery vehicles: chewing gum, skin patches, lozenges and nasal spray.

There are drugs available on prescription (but not by dentists) that are effective in helping smokers stop smoking. **Bupropion** (Zyban) works by blocking nicotinic receptors and thus reduces the craving for nicotine. A side effect of this medication, which was originally used as an antidepressant, is dryness of the mouth. **Varenicline (Champix)** prevents nicotine from reaching nicotine receptors in the brain and also stimulates dopamine production, both of which make cigarette smoking less satisfying.

Smoking-cessation services

Across the United Kingdom a range of smoking-cessation services have been established to help smokers give up (Table 32.1). These services provide interactive websites and telephone helplines.

Unproven aids to stopping smoking

Acupuncture

A recent Cochrane systematic review found no evidence that acupuncture or associated acupressure was helpful in assisting smokers to quit, but noted that a lack of consistent evidence meant that no firm conclusions could be drawn. Although safe when correctly applied, acupuncture is likely to be less effective than current evidence-based interventions in helping smokers give up.

Hypnotherapy

Hypnotherapy has been widely promoted as an aid to smoking cessation. The theory is that hypnosis can be used to strengthen the resolve to quit, or to weaken the desire to smoke. There is not enough evidence to know whether hypnotherapy could be as effective as straightforward counselling.

The role of the dental team in providing smoking-cessation advice

Members of the dental team are in an ideal position to identify patients who smoke and who are contemplating giving up. Dentists are often the only healthcare professionals who see healthy young adults who are smokers on a regular basis. Smoking status should form a core question in taking a patient's medical history. This can act as a prompt to discussing the effects of smoking on oral health. The role of the dental team has been described using the '4As' as an aide mémoire (Table 32.2).

Having identified patients who are interested in stopping smoking, dentists should refer them to the local smoking-cessation services, who have the expertise to provide appropriate counselling and can prescribe effective medication to help overcome nicotine withdrawal. Given the cyclical nature of smoking-cessation attempts, it is useful to enquire about progress at subsequent appointments. ***Smokefree and Smiling***, a leaflet produced by the Department of Health in England, provides a helpful guide to the role of the dental team in activities related to smoking cessation.

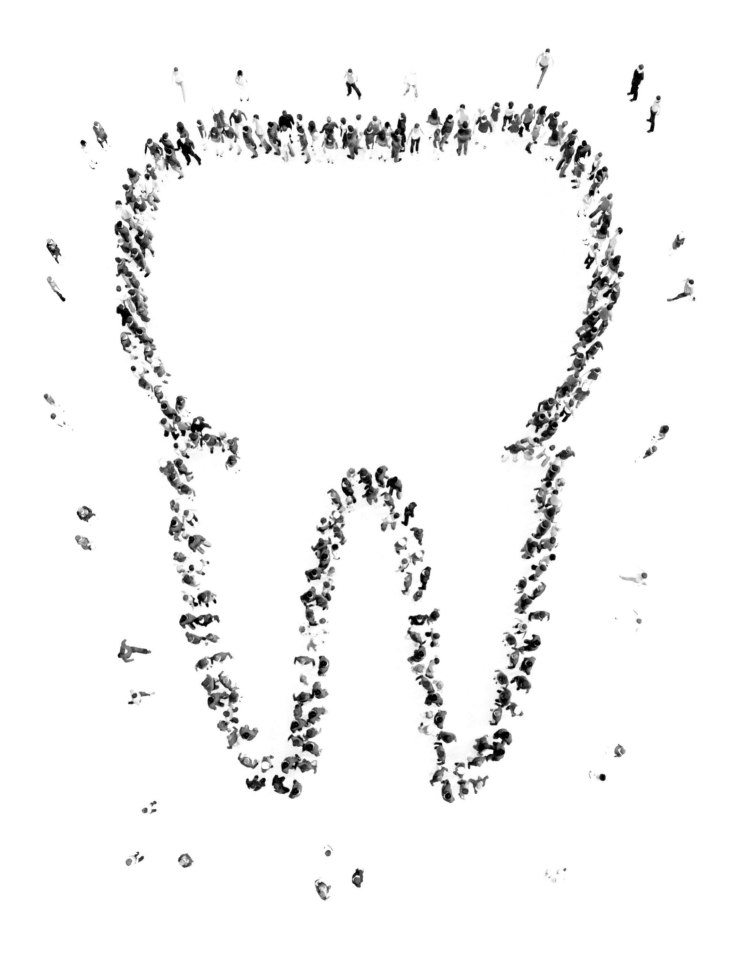

Alcohol and oral health

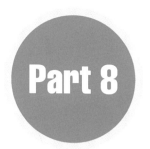

Part 8

33 Alcohol and oral health

Figure 33.1 Impact of alcohol on oral heath and dentistry

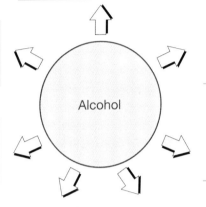

Alcohol is a risk factor for oral cancer

Management of patients with alcohol induced health problems, e.g. reduced clotting times

Trauma to oral and facial tissues can occur when patients are drunk

Dental professionals themselves may be at risk from excess use of alcohol

Consumption of excess alcoholic drinks of low pH (e.g. wine) can result in non-carious tooth surface loss - as can gastric reflux associated with alcohol abuse

Alcohol

Dentists and their team may, by providing brief advice, make patients aware of their alcohol consumption

Dental professionals can identify people with potentially harmful patterns of alcohol consumption when taking a medical history

Table 33.1 Recommended safe limits of alcohol consumption

Gender	Guidance
Men	Should drink **no more than 21 units of alcohol per week**, no more than 4 units in any one day and have at least two alcohol-free days per week.
Women	Should drink **no more than 14 units of alcohol per week**, no more than 3 units in any one day and have at least two alcohol-free days per week.
Pregnant women	Pregnant women or women who are trying to conceive **should not drink alcohol at all**. If they insist on drinking, then to minimize the risk to the unborn child, they should not drink more than 1–2 units of alcohol once or twice a week and should not get drunk at all.
Definition of a unit of alcohol	**1 unit = 10 ml by volume or 8 g by weight of pure alcohol**
Examples	
1 unit of alcohol	One half pint of ordinary-strength beer, lager or cider (3–4% ABV)
1 unit of alcohol	Small pub measure of spirits – 25 ml (40% ABV)
1.5 units of alcohol	Small glass (125 ml) wine (ABV 12%)
3 units of alcohol	One half litre (500 ml, just under a pint) of strong beer (6% ABV)
3.5 units of alcohol	Large glass (250 ml) wine (ABV 14%)

Box 33.1 Health complications of excess alcohol consumption

Liver disease (cirrhosis or hepatitis)
Cancer
Gut and pancreas disorders
Depression
Anxiety
Sexual difficulties
Hypertension
Accidents/trauma
Obesity

Alcohol and health

The consumption of alcohol is an integral part of the social fabric of most developed and many developing countries. While alcohol is a legal commodity, consumption of more than a defined maximum has adverse impacts on health, as well as economic and social circumstances. In the United Kingdom, the prescribed safe alcohol consumption limits are as shown in Table 33.1. The Alcohol Health Alliance, which represents 44 organizations committed to reducing the damage caused to health by alcohol misuse, reports that every year in the United Kingdom, 1 million hospital admissions are related to alcohol and alcohol accounts for 10% of the burden of disease and death. The government estimates that alcohol-related harm currently costs the National Health Service £3.7 billion every year (equal to £120 for every tax payer) and wider UK society more than £21 billion – more than double the £10 billion revenue generated from alcohol taxes.

Surveys show that a large proportion of the population routinely exceed the recommended limits. Excess consumption occurs in two main ways: long-term regular (daily) exposure to alcohol; and binge drinking, where the safe levels of consumption are regularly exceeded, interspersed with periods of no or limited drinking. The latter pattern of consumption has been particularly common in young people in the United Kingdom in recent years. Some people's consumption of alcohol reaches a stage where they become addicted and on a journey that often results in them losing everything in their life and eventually life itself; they are termed alcoholics. The common diseases related to excess alcohol consumption are shown in Box 33.1.

In addition to the impact on health, alcohol-related crime, disorder and domestic violence are significant social consequences of alcohol misuse.

Alcohol and dentistry

Alcohol can have impacts on dentistry and oral health in a number of ways (Figure 33.1). It is a well-recognized risk factor for oral cancer, particularly in combination with smoking tobacco. Alcohol can also affect treatment, either by causing oral-facial trauma, by leading to systemic disease (e.g. liver disease) that complicates patient management, or when patients present for treatment under the influence of alcohol. Alcohol-reduction advice by dental professionals is discussed shortly.

Dentistry is recognized as a potentially stressful occupation and recourse to alcohol use in excess is an occupational hazard. Members of the dental team have a duty to be aware of their own alcohol consumption and to watch out for signs of alcohol abuse in colleagues and employees.

Actions to reduce alcohol misuse

At a population level

Upstream actions to reduce alcohol misuse vary from country to country. For instance, in Scandinavia the sale of alcohol is very strictly controlled and it can only be purchased from special points of sale. In other countries alcohol is readily available, too readily available in the view of many healthcare professionals. While legislation exists to prohibit the sale of alcohol to minors, there is great concern at the ease with which this can be circumvented, enabling teenagers and adolescents to access alcohol.

Currently, there is a great political debate in the United Kingdom over the introduction of a **minimum unit price** for alcohol. Advocates for public health suggest that this will curb the sale of cheap high-strength alcoholic drinks by supermarkets and corner shops – often suspected as the sources of alcohol purchased by or on behalf of minors. Opponents argue that rather than legislate for a minimum alcohol unit price, it is preferable to work with the drinks industry to achieve agreement on the pricing and marketing of alcohol, particularly to young people and adolescents, by responsible advertising and drinks promotions.

This is a good illustration of the concept of the '**nanny state**'. A perennial problem for public health is to what extent government should legislate to influence and control people's lifestyles and life circumstances, or whether this should be left to market and other forces to decide. Obviously, a sensible balance needs to be struck between over-regulation for health and a free-for-all, where people fail to act in their own best interests or in those of fellow members of society.

At an individual level

It has also been suggested that as part of their overall holistic care of patients, members of the dental team are in a good position to identify those who are consuming more than the safe level of alcohol. The argument is that dentists, therapists and hygienists see fit and healthy patients who may not otherwise have routine contact with a healthcare professional. While dentist involvement in alcohol-related advice has been explored in the context of drunk patients attending Accident and Emergency departments with facial injuries, the potential for dentists to get involved in alcohol-reduction advice in dental practice has yet to be fully investigated. It certainly has not been considered to the same extent as dentists' involvement in smoking-cessation advice.

Screening questions on a medical history form may highlight a patient with excess alcohol consumption. The Fast Alcohol Screening Test (FAST) is a way of identifying those whose alcohol intake is a cause for concern. Giving brief motivational advice and 'maximizing the teachable moment' is held as an important action to help patients moderate their alcohol intake. An example is where a patient who has been involved in an alcohol-inspired fight requires stitches for facial trauma. When they return to have their wound checked and are sober and have had the chance to reflect on the events that led to their injury, they may be susceptible to brief alcohol-reduction advice.

The key current issues in this regard are the degree to which dental practitioners feel prepared to ask patients about their drinking, and whether they are properly equipped to advise patients identified as in need of alcohol-reduction advice and to make the necessary onward referral to the patient's general medical practitioner. In addition, patients' expectations of being asked about their drinking when attending a dental professional may be a further issue.

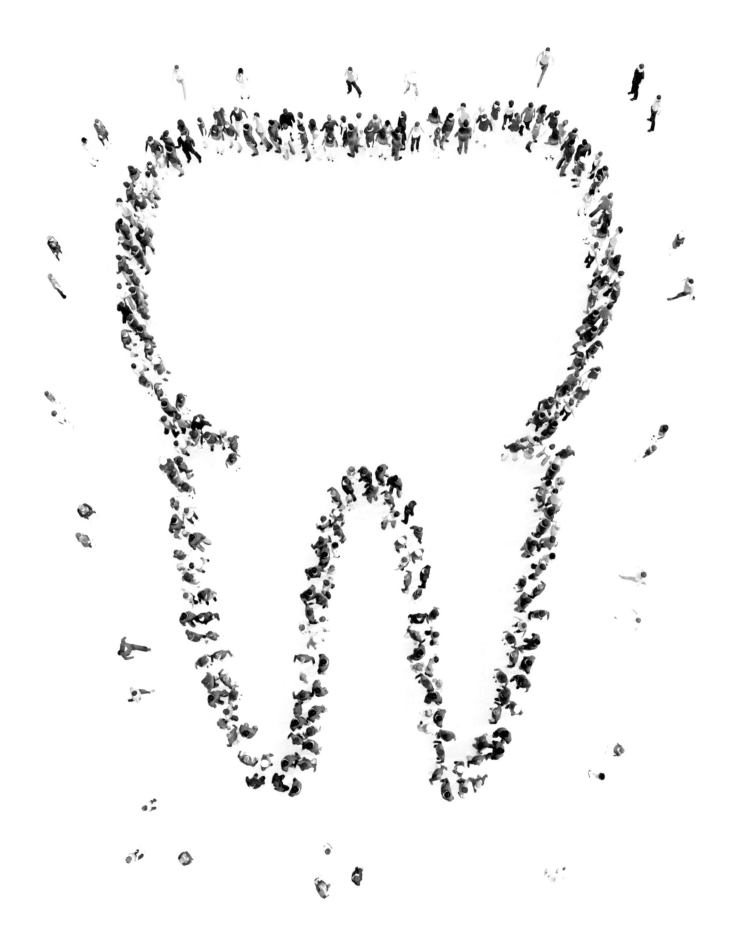

Assessing health needs

Part 9

Chapters

34 Assessing oral health needs on a population basis

Figure 34.1 Information requirements in health needs assessment and service planning

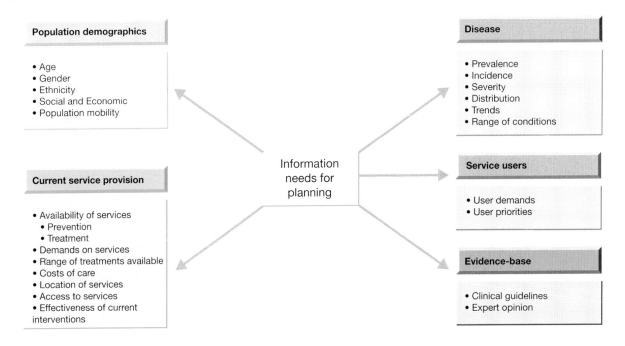

Population demographics
- Age
- Gender
- Ethnicity
- Social and Economic
- Population mobility

Current service provision
- Availability of services
  - Prevention
  - Treatment
- Demands on services
- Range of treatments available
- Costs of care
- Location of services
- Access to services
- Effectiveness of current interventions

Information needs for planning

Disease
- Prevalence
- Incidence
- Severity
- Distribution
- Trends
- Range of conditions

Service users
- User demands
- User priorities

Evidence-base
- Clinical guidelines
- Expert opinion

Figure 34.2 Relationship between health needs, demand, supply and influencing factors

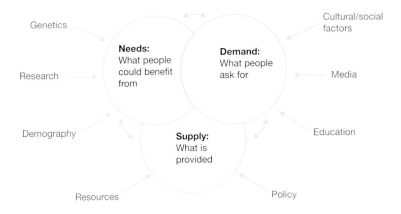

Genetics

Cultural/social factors

Needs: What people could benefit from

Demand: What people ask for

Research

Media

Demography

Supply: What is provided

Education

Resources

Policy

Figure 34.3 Where needs assessment fits into the planning cycle

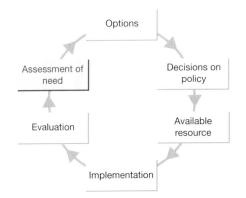

Options

Assessment of need

Decisions on policy

Evaluation

Available resource

Implementation

Dental Public Health at a Glance, First Edition. Ivor G. Chestnutt.
© 2016 John Wiley & Sons, Ltd. Published 2016 by John Wiley & Sons, Ltd.

Determining oral health needs

For an individual patient

When treating a patient in a clinical setting, a dentist will gather facts about the individual by asking questions and undertaking a clinical examination. The information gathered, possibly supplemented by special tests or investigations, will enable the dentist to make a diagnosis of the patient's condition. In consultation with the patient, the dentist will be able to assess the patient's needs and discuss treatment options, from which a treatment plan can be formulated and agreed. This process is known as **diagnosis and treatment planning**.

For a population

In dental public health a similar process occurs, although instead of considering the needs of an individual patient, a public health dentist has to consider the needs of a population, or subgroup within a population. This process is known as **oral health needs assessment**.

Oral health needs assessment

Oral health needs assessment involves:

- Examining and describing the characteristics of the population.
- Identifying their needs, including taking into account the wishes of the population.
- Examining current service provision and its capacity to meet the needs of the population.
- Where gaps exist, identifying how these can be met, either by reorganizing existing services, investing in new services or decommissioning services that are no longer required or fit for purpose.

The purpose of oral health needs assessment is to:

- Identify and quantify oral health needs.
- Identify potential health gains.
- Permit prioritization of identified needs.
- Inform the planning and commissioning of oral health services.

An understanding of how to assess oral health needs is therefore a fundamental component of dental public health practice.

How to conduct an oral health needs assessment

Needs can be viewed from different perspectives, such as normative/expressed/felt/comparative need, as discussed in Chapter 40.

Needs assessment can also be conducted from a range of perspectives:

- **Epidemiological**
  - Disease prevalence/incidence in distinct geographical localities, e.g. caries prevalence in different local authority areas.
  - Specific diseases, e.g. oral cancer incidence in older men from disadvantaged backgrounds.
- **Comparative**
  - Comparing services/providers in different localities, e.g. waiting lists for orthodontic treatment.
- **Corporate**
  - Draws on the views of different groups, e.g. providers of healthcare on the provision of oral care for nursing home residents, local people on the provision of out-of-hours dental care.

Information used in health needs planning is shown in Figure 34.1.

Need, demand and supply

In addition to **need**, there are two other factors that have to be considered when planning and delivering a health service. These are **demand** and **supply**.

Need is what people could benefit from, for instance greater provision of NHS dentistry in a given area.

Demand is what people want, such as easier access to NHS dentistry, expressed perhaps by letters of complaint to local public representatives.

Supply is what is provided, for example the existing number of dentists accepting patients for NHS care.

The relationship between health needs, demand and supply and the factors that influence them are shown in Figure 34.2.

The planning cycle

Health service planning should ideally be a cyclical process, where needs assessment forms a vital role in informing the options available. However, the process of planning is often constrained by the resources available and by political influences on health service provision. The place of health needs assessment in the planning cycle is shown in Figure 34.3.

The role of local authorities in service planning

Joint strategic needs assessment

The Health and Social Care Act 2012 in England transferred much of the responsibility for public health from the National Health Service to local authorities. Planning in local authorities is undertaken by Health and Wellbeing Boards (HWBs), which were also established by this Act. Their decision making is guided by a joint strategic needs assessment (JSNA). This is defined as a process that identifies current and future health and wellbeing needs in the light of existing services and informs future service planning, taking into account evidence of effectiveness. A JSNA identifies the 'big picture', in terms of the health and wellbeing needs and inequalities of a local population. Producing a JSNA is a mandatory requirement designed to help organizations with service planning and the commissioning process.

Health and Wellbeing Boards

Health and Wellbeing Boards are designed as a forum where health and social care work together to improve the health and wellbeing of their local population and reduce health inequalities. Each top-tier and unitary authority has its own HWB. The membership of HWBs is mandated in law and includes a local elected representative (councillor), senior staff from the local authority and clinical commissioning groups and the Director of Public Health.

In Wales, Health Boards and local government have a joint statutory duty to develop a Health, Social Care and Wellbeing Strategy. This focuses on:

- Improving health and wellbeing and reducing inequalities.
- The provision, quality, integration and sustainability of services that are provided jointly by health and social services, e.g. nursing, care and residential homes.

In Scotland affirmative action is underway to integrate health and social care. A schedule of expected outcomes at the overlap between health and social care has been established by the Scottish government.

35 The oral health needs of specific population groups

Table 35.1 Special care dentistry

Special Care Dentistry (SCD)

Special Care Dentistry (SCD) is recognized as a distinct dental specialty. Dentists with appropriate postgraduate training and experience can apply to the General Dental Council (GDC) for entry to the Specialist List in SCD. The GDC describes SCD as 'providing preventive and treatment oral care services for adults who are unable to accept routine dental care because of some physical, intellectual, medical, emotional, sensory, mental or social impairment, or a combination of these factors'.

Table 35.2 Prison dentistry

Prison Dentistry

Responsibility for commissioning of prison dental services now lies with the NHS, while in the past prison services contracted directly with dental providers. Providing dental care for prisoners poses a number of challenges.

Issues include:
- Prisoners' oral health is among the poorest in any group. The majority of prisoners come from areas of low social and economic status and their oral health is said to be four times worse than that of their peers.
- Prisoners have significant general health issues that can complicate their dental management. These include poor mental health, illegal drug use, and dependency on alcohol and tobacco.
- Prior to imprisonment many prisoners are sporadic dental attenders, many attending only when in pain.
- Implementation of oral hygiene regimes in prison needs to account for potential security issues to prevent oral hygiene aids being used as weapons.
- Most prisons have an in-house dental surgery, but the efficiency of dental services can be low, with only a few prisoners being seen in each treatment session. This can be attributed to the need for prisoners to be escorted to the prison dental surgery; organizational issues meaning that prison officers need to be available to escort the prisoners to the surgery from their cell; and patients refusing to attend at the last minute.
- A 2014 survey has shown that much of the clinical infrastructure in prisons is outdated and in need of modernization.
- Many prisoners are anxious about dental treatment, having had limited exposure to dental care prior to incarceration.
- The transient nature of the prison population: prisoners move from remand to longer-term prisons; prisoners are moved from one institution to another; and the short terms that many prisoners serve mean that completing a course of treatment can be problematic.

Table 35.3 Armed forces dentistry

Armed Forces Dentisty

The military form a distinct group within the population whose dental care needs require special consideration.

In the United Kingdom, dental care for soldiers, sailors, airmen and their families is provided by the Defence Dental Service (DDS). The DDS is a tri-service organization employing around 1085 personnel from the Royal Navy, Army, Royal Air Force and civilian sector who are trained dentists, hygienists, technicians or dental nurses, as well as critical support staff. Most treatment is provided at service establishments (dental centres) in the United Kingdom and in centres where the British military are permanently deployed – Cyprus and Germany. Military dentists are appointed as officers and undergo 14 weeks' basic military training before their first posting. A limited number of cadetships are available to dental students in the United Kingdom.

There are a number of specific issues in providing care for military personnel:
- A high level of oral fitness needs to be secured for military personnel before they are deployed on operational tours of duty. Oral health is viewed as an important element of overall medical fitness for duty.
- Two groups of military personnel require especially good attention to oral health:
  - Submariners – who may be at sea for months at a time.
  - Jet pilots – the high gravitational forces experienced while flying lead to barometric changes that can result in toothache in moribund pulp chambers, around leaking restorations.
- Many of the young men and women recruited to the infantry come from low social and economic circumstances and may have higher disease experience as a result. They require an intensive course of dental treatment to make them dentally fit and thus fit for service.

Specific population groups

In society there are groups who share common characteristics that require particular consideration in the commissioning and organization of dental care.

People with physical and mental disabilities

Many people with physical and mental disabilities will be able to undergo routine dental care in the General Dental Service. However, those whose disabilities are more severe may require care from a clinician experienced in the provision of special/additional care (Table 35.1). Such patients are frequently cared for by the Community (Salaried/Public) Dental Service. For those patients who require care using general anaesthesia, admission to the Hospital Dental Service may be required. The British Society for Disability and Oral Health has issued guidelines for the care of those with physical and mental disabilities.

Issues include:
* Prevention – providing appropriately tailored primary prevention.
* Physical access to surgeries (for wheelchairs/steps/stairs).
* The availability of specialized equipment, e.g. hoists to lift patients into the dental chair, equipment that can recline the patient's own wheelchair, a bariatric chair (to accommodate patients whose body weight exceeds the capacity of a conventional dental chair).
* Access to general anaesthetic/conscious sedation services.
* Knowledge of and compliance with the requirements of the Mental Capacity Act 2005 to ensure valid consent.
* Making certain that patients are managed in a holistic fashion, to ensure that their dental care is integrated into other complex needs.

Frail elderly people

The increased number of older people, the majority of whom will increasingly have their own teeth (Chapter 9), merit consideration as a specific population group, particularly the frail elderly. These people are often resident in care homes and are dependent on others for many, if not all, aspects of daily living.

Issues include:
* As more old people retain their own teeth, the need to ensure adequate oral hygiene will assume increasing importance. This will necessitate education for carers in how to provide this.
* An individual oral health needs assessment should be undertaken for all people on admission to residential care facilities.
* Mobility – frail elderly people may be house or bed bound and unable to travel to a dental surgery for care. This requires domiciliary care. Here the dentist travels to the patient, as opposed to the more usual patient coming to see the dentist.
* Mobile dental equipment – improved equipment including high-torque handpieces makes bedside care more feasible.
* Difficulty tolerating treatment.
* Lack of mental capacity and the need to adhere to legal requirements to ensure consent is valid and treatment is in the patient's best interest when they lack understanding of their own care needs.
* Co-morbidity:
  * dental problems may have an impact on general health
  * general health, and the medications used to treat problems, may have an impact on oral health.
* Many care homes have arrangements with local general dental practitioners to provide care for their residents. Changes to the NHS Contract in 2006 reduced the availability of domiciliary care and now such arrangements frequently have to be made on an independent/private basis. Some Community Dental Services

have established **managed clinical networks** to administer domiciliary care.
* Social enterprise companies are a possible means of addressing the provision of dental care to care homes.

Homeless people

The homeless are those who lack permanent accommodation. Homeless people may be living in temporary accommodation, bed-and-breakfast establishments or hostels, 'sofa-surfing', staying with friends or sleeping rough. In late 2014, there were just under 61,000 households in England accepted by local authorities as officially homeless. It is estimated that in England, 2400 people sleep rough each night. Access to healthcare is a significant issue for people who are homeless. Surveys show that access to dental care comes high on the list of health needs of people living on the streets.

Issues include:
* Levels of decay and tooth loss are higher than in the general population.
* Older homeless people are frequently edentulous and do not have dentures.
* Homeless people lack social and supportive contacts.
* Mental health issues compound other problems.
* Addiction to alcohol and drugs is common, leading to further dental health problems.

Gypsies and Travellers

Gypsies and Travellers are a specific cultural group who are vulnerable and frequently experience difficulty in accessing dental care. Data on their oral health needs are limited to non-existent. This group is frequently invisible to Commissioners, not only in relation to oral health but health in general.

Issues include:
* They frequently live in overcrowded and less than satisfactory accommodation.
* Levels of disease are higher and life expectancy is lower than in the general population.
* Cultural beliefs affect their trust in health professionals.
* They face racism and prejudice.
* Their access to healthcare is problematic.
* Their levels of general literacy and health literacy are low.

Substance misusers

The following issues have impacts on oral health and dental care for people who are addicted to drugs and alcohol:
* They experience high levels of dental caries, which is untreated.
* Their chaotic lifestyle prevents routine dental attendance and they may fail to keep appointments.
* Patients are likely to present in acute dental pain.
* Patients may have significant health problems, such as blood-borne virus infection, mental health issues.
* Addicts may demand opiate-based analgesics, e.g. codeine.
* Methadone, used in heroin-replacement therapy programmes, is cariogenic due to its high sugar content – the sugar-free variety should be encouraged.

Other groups

Two specific groups who have special arrangements for the provision of dental care are the armed forces and prisoners. Issues related to these groups are shown in Tables 35.2 and 35.3.

36 Screening and diagnostic tests

Figure 36.1 The parameters that can be calculated to determine the value of a screening or diagnostic test

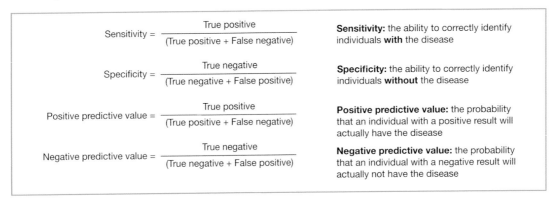

$$\text{Sensitivity} = \frac{\text{True positive}}{(\text{True positive} + \text{False negative})}$$

Sensitivity: the ability to correctly identify individuals **with** the disease

$$\text{Specificity} = \frac{\text{True negative}}{(\text{True negative} + \text{False positive})}$$

Specificity: the ability to correctly identify individuals **without** the disease

$$\text{Positive predictive value} = \frac{\text{True positive}}{(\text{True positive} + \text{False negative})}$$

Positive predictive value: the probability that an individual with a positive result will actually have the disease

$$\text{Negative predictive value} = \frac{\text{True negative}}{(\text{True negative} + \text{False positive})}$$

Negative predictive value: the probability that an individual with a negative result will actually not have the disease

Figure 36.2 Diagrammatic representation of a receiver operating diagnostic (ROC) curve

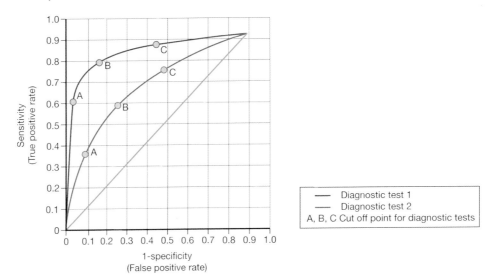

Sensitivity (True positive rate) vs 1-specificity (False positive rate)

— Diagnostic test 1
— Diagnostic test 2
A, B, C Cut off point for diagnostic tests

Table 36.1 Criteria for the establishment of a screening programme

Criteria	Considerations
Is the disease an important health issue?	The prevalence and impact of the disease require consideration.
Is the screening test acceptable to patients?	If the screening test is overly burdensome or in some way is not acceptable to the majority of the population to be screened, uptake will be low and the programme ineffective.
Is there a recognizable latent or early symptomatic stage?	There is little point screening for a disease that will, at an early stage, become evident and lead the patient to seek care due to signs and symptoms.
Are facilities for diagnosis and treatment available?	A positive screen will require the resources to undertake a definitive diagnostic test and to treat patients confirmed as having the disease.
Has the opportunity cost been considered?	Spending money and resources on a screening programme means that these resources are not available to use for an alternative intervention.
Is there an agreed policy on who to treat as patients?	This means is it clear when an individual has the disease and when not – is a definitive diagnosis possible?
Does treatment confer benefit?	This raises the question of whether there is any material advantage to the patient in identifying their disease earlier than would otherwise be the case. If knowing the patient has the disease early results in a better health outcome, then clearly screening is advantageous. However, if there is no difference in treatment outcome as a result of early diagnosis, then a screening programme may add unnecessarily to costs and result in patients having longer knowledge of the disease with no material benefit, and the possible worry of knowing they have the disease and being labelled as a patient.

Source: *Wilson and Jinger 1968. Reproduced with permission from World Health Organization.*

Dental Public Health at a Glance, First Edition. Ivor G. Chestnutt.
© 2016 John Wiley & Sons, Ltd. Published 2016 by John Wiley & Sons, Ltd.

Screening

Screening in the context of public health programmes is usually designed to enable early diagnosis of a disease or condition.

Screening implies the systematic application of a test or procedure to a population perceived to be at risk of the disease of interest.

Examples of screening programmes in the United Kingdom are the range of tests applied to all newborn babies to detect metabolic disorders, and programmes to detect breast and cervical cancer in women and bowel cancer in both men and women. There are no formal national screening programmes for oral disease.

Screening versus diagnosis

It is very important to understand the difference between screening and diagnosis. Screening aims to identify those who are likely to have the disease in question. A positive screening test does not always imply that the individual has the disease. Often further, more definitive or invasive tests are required to confirm diagnosis. So in the case of screening for bowel cancer, a positive occult blood sample in a stool sample requires further investigation to determine whether cancer is present.

Criteria for the establishment of a screening programme

There are a number of criteria that need to be satisfied before a screening programme is implemented (Table 36.1).

Oral cancer

Recommendations on the implementation of a screening programme for a given disease are made by the UK National Screening Committee. When oral cancer was last reviewed, the committee concluded that systematic population screening was not justified. Instead, current practice is for dental professionals to undertake opportunistic screening.

Dental caries

For most of the twentieth century the Community Dental Service (and its predecessor the School Dental Service) undertook 'school dental screening' and there was a statutory obligation to do so. While this process was called screening, it was in fact diagnosis. The objective of the exercise was to identify children who had untreated dental decay and who were not under the care of a dentist, and to inform parents of their child's oral status. In the latter part of the twentieth century, the effectiveness of mass screening of school children for dental decay was questioned. The main issue was, once the need was identified, ensuring that parents subsequently took children to the dentist. The role of the Community Dental Service changed from routine care of children to focusing on looking after those with special needs. This has led to traditional school screening being abandoned in most areas.

The value of a screening or diagnostic test

The application of a diagnostic or screening test can have four possible outcomes, as shown in Table 36.2. The usefulness of a screening or diagnostic test is dependent on the proportion of individuals who have the disease and are correctly identified as having the disease in question (**sensitivity**) and the proportion of individuals who do not have the disease and are correctly identified as not having the disease (**specificity**); see Figure 36.1. Clearly, it is desirable to have both of these proportions as high as possible. They are influenced by the cut-off point for the screening or diagnostic test in question. Increasing the cut-off point to increase the sensitivity of a test results in a decrease in its specificity. So setting up the test to increase the proportion of people who are correctly tested as positive means that there is a trade-off in the number of individuals correctly identified as not having the disease.

Receiver operating characteristic (ROC) curves

The usefulness of a screening or diagnostic test can be demonstrated visually by plotting a receiver operating characteristic (ROC) curve, as shown in Figure 36.2.

Examples of the use of ROC curves in dentistry include the evaluation of tests determining caries risk in children; histological validation of cone-beam computed tomography versus laser fluorescence and conventional diagnostic methods for occlusal caries detection; and validating screening methods for periodontitis using salivary haemoglobin level and self-report questionnaires in disabled people.

The sensitivity (true positive rate) is plotted against 1-sensitivity (the false positive rate) for different cut-off points used to define positive and negative in the test (e.g. points A, B and C on Figure 36.2). A diagonal line is drawn at 45 degrees through the origin. The area under the curve to this line relates to the performance of the test. So the further the curve approaches the top left of the graph, the better the test. In Figure 36.2, Test 1 (red line) has greater utility (i.e. is better at correctly identifying positives and negatives) than Test 2 (blue line).

Table 36.2 The possible outcomes from the application of a screening or diagnostic test

Test result	Disease status	
	Has the disease	Does not have the disease
Positive	True positive	False positive
Negative	False negative	True negative

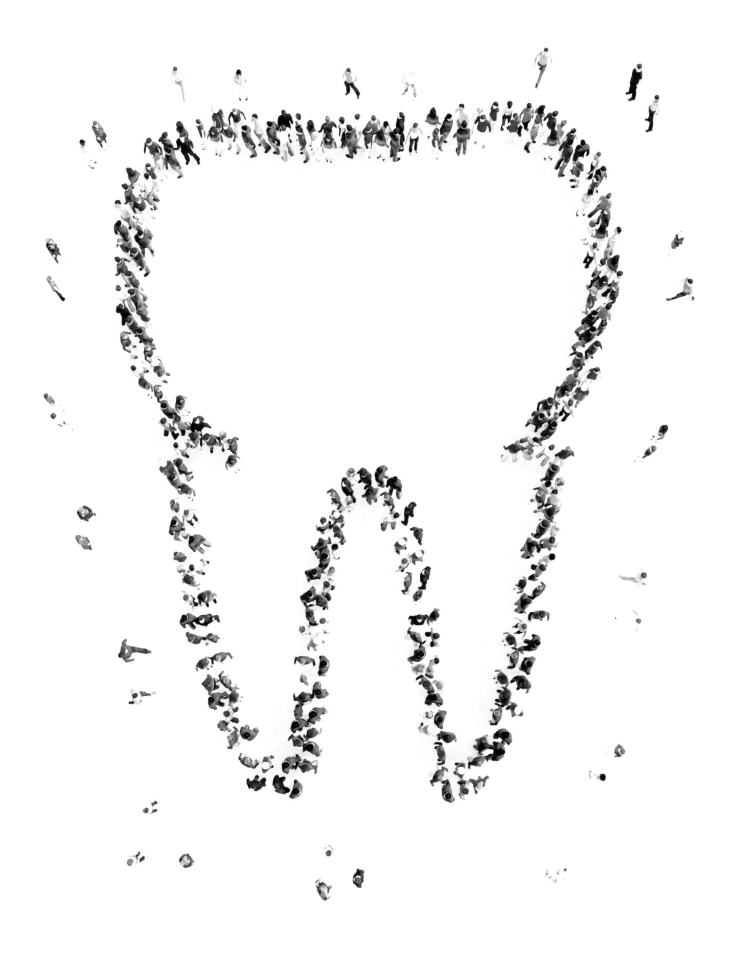

Providing dental services

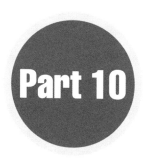

Part 10

Chapters

37 Health economics

Table 37.1 Approaches to health economic analysis

Cost-Minimization Analysis

When to use	Dental example	Notes
Cost-minimization analysis is used when the health outcomes of two or more interventions are the same or very similar in all important aspects – and have been shown to be so in a clinical trial.	This type of analysis would be suitable to evaluate the use of two mouthwashes that resulted in the same level of dental plaque reduction and had similar side-effect profiles. It could be used in comparing a branded product with a generic version of the same product. The least costly option would be that of choice.	This a simple technique, but requires the data to confirm that the clinical and side-effect outcomes are the same.

Cost–Utility Analysis

When to use	Dental example	Notes
Cost–utility analysis is used to compare different interventions with varying health outcomes. The common 'currency' of a utility measure, most commonly a QUALY, is used to compare outcomes.	This type of analysis would be suitable to evaluate different approaches to the treatment of head and neck cancer.	It is necessary to define and measure the health states of interest. The utility can be considered either from the perspective of individual patients or society. Techniques for eliciting utility values include: • Standard gamble • Time trade-off • Visual analogue or rating scale.

Cost-Effectiveness Analysis

When to use	Dental example	Notes
Cost-effectiveness analysis is used when the health benefits of interventions are measured in natural units, reflecting a dominant common therapeutic goal for different therapies.	This type of analysis could be used to compare the relative merits of fissure sealants and fluoride varnish in the prevention of new caries lesions on the occlusal surfaces of teeth. Here the unit of analysis is the number of carious surfaces avoided.	Results would be presented in the form of how much it costs to prevent an additional tooth surface from becoming carious (incremental cost). The different interventions are compared by determining the cost-effectiveness ratio. This is calculated by diving the cost of the intervention by the health effect outcome. This is the most common type of health economic analysis reported in the literature.

Cost–Benefit Analysis

When to use	Dental example	Notes
Cost–benefit analysis is used when both costs and benefits are measured in monetary units. The financial value of the costs are compared with the financial benefits of the interventions.	Cost–benefit analysis has been used to determine the economic impact of water fluoridation.	The intervention is deemed favourable when the financial value of the benefits is in excess of the financial value of the costs. This approach does not take into account quality-of-life measurements and thus is unable to account for different patient groups with different outcome measures. This approach informs value for money and can guide priority setting.

Dental Public Health at a Glance, First Edition. Ivor G. Chestnutt.
© 2016 John Wiley & Sons, Ltd. Published 2016 by John Wiley & Sons, Ltd.

Health economics

Health economics deals with scarcity of resources and the clinical effectiveness and cost effectiveness of healthcare provision. Health economic analysis informs how maximum value can be achieved from the resources available.

Maximizing outcome from scarce resources

The resources available to provide healthcare, whether viewed from the perspective of an individual, a health insurance company or a government, are finite. The potential needs for and potential to benefit from healthcare are infinite. In the United Kingdom, the population is increasing in number and ageing. Medical and dental technology is ever expanding in both scope and complexity. Society and those who make decisions on its behalf therefore face the difficult decision of how the defined resources available are best used to achieve the optimum outcome.

Typical decisions facing politicians, health policy makers and clinicians are as follows. If a new drug for treating cancer costs £40,000 per patient cared for, is that a better use of the money than providing joint replacements costing £10,000 each for four patients? In coming to a decision on this matter, it is necessary not only to consider the number of patients treated, but the clinical outcome and the quality of life resulting for the patients concerned. If the cancer drug extends the patient's life by six months but the joint replacement relieves pain, increases mobility and lasts for ten years, which is the better use of the £40,000?

These are the types of question that health economics helps answer, because resources are always **scarce**. This means that both the **clinical effectiveness** and **cost effectiveness** of interventions have to be considered when planning and commissioning resources. The following concepts are important in health economics.

Clinical effectiveness

As is evident from the name, clinical effectiveness relates to the clinical/health outcome of an intervention. It is about what works and is central to the concept of evidence-based practice (Chapter 18).

Cost effectiveness

Cost effectiveness implies either a desire to achieve a predetermined objective at least cost, or a desire to maximize the benefit to the population of patients served from a limited amount of resources.

Efficiency

Efficiency evaluates how well resources are used to achieve a desired outcome.

Utility measures

Utility is defined as the level of satisfaction that consumers derive from having their desires met. In the context of health economics, it relates to preferences for different health states. Utility measures have two dimensions – a quantitative dimension, which measures enhanced survival (years added to life), and a qualitative dimension, which accounts for the quality of life (QoL, life added to years). Quality of life is assessed using components such as ability to perform the functions of daily living, presence of pain and mental disturbance.

Quality-adjusted life years (QALYs)

The years added to life by a health intervention and the quality of life during those years are combined to produce a QALY. This reflects the number of years lived in a given health state. QALYs are presented as a value between 0 and 1, where 0 = death and 1 = one year of life in perfect health. A score less than 0 would indicate a health state worse than death. The advantage of this approach is that it allows health interventions with different clinical outcomes to be compared, as in the example of the new cancer drug and the provision of joint replacements given earlier.

The costs of different health interventions can be expressed as the cost per QALY gained. For publicly funded health interventions, the National Institute for Health and Care Excellence (NICE) currently values one QALY at between £20,000 and £30,000.

QALYs and oral health

The application of analysis using QALYs to oral health interventions is problematic, as dental procedures generally are not directly life lengthening. The concept of **quality-adjusted tooth years (QATYs)**, where a missing tooth would score 0 and a sound functioning tooth would score 1, has been proposed, but has not been used to any great degree.

Types of health economic evaluation

There are four common types of economic evaluation:
- Cost-minimization analysis
- Cost–utility analysis
- Cost-effectiveness analysis
- Cost–benefit analysis

These are described in Table 37.1. The frequency with which these analyses are described in the economic analysis of caries-prevention programmes is shown in Table 37.2.

Capital and recurrent costs

In health service planning, costs are described as capital and recurrent. Capital costs are one-off costs that are not directly linked to output. Typical examples are equipment, for instance a dental chair, an autoclave, a new surgery. Recurrent costs, as the name suggests, represent expenditure that is repeated and on-going, such as staff salaries, materials, costs of using equipment such as electricity, annual service charges.

In any healthcare system staff costs (salaries) are usually the largest item of expenditure, consuming about 40% of the NHS budget in England.

Opportunity costs

Because resources are finite, there is an **opportunity cost** to all decisions in healthcare. This means that if we decide to undertake activity *x*, then we are required to forego activity *y*. As an example, if a dental practice owner decides to spend one hour each month holding a staff meeting, that time cannot be used to see and treat patients. The opportunity cost of the meeting is reduced patient throughput. However, in the interests of an efficiently run and safe practice, it is likely that the benefit of the staff meeting will outweigh not treating patients during that one-hour session and the reduction in income that results.

Table 37.2 Frequency of different health economic approaches observed in a systematic review of economic evaluations of caries prevention programmes

Type of economic analysis	Number reported
Cost-effectiveness analysis	30
Cost–benefit analysis	22
Cost-effectiveness and cost–benefit analysis	5
Cost–utility analysis	5
Cost-minimization analysis	2

Source: *Data from Marino et al. 2013.*

38 How dental care is organized in the United Kingdom

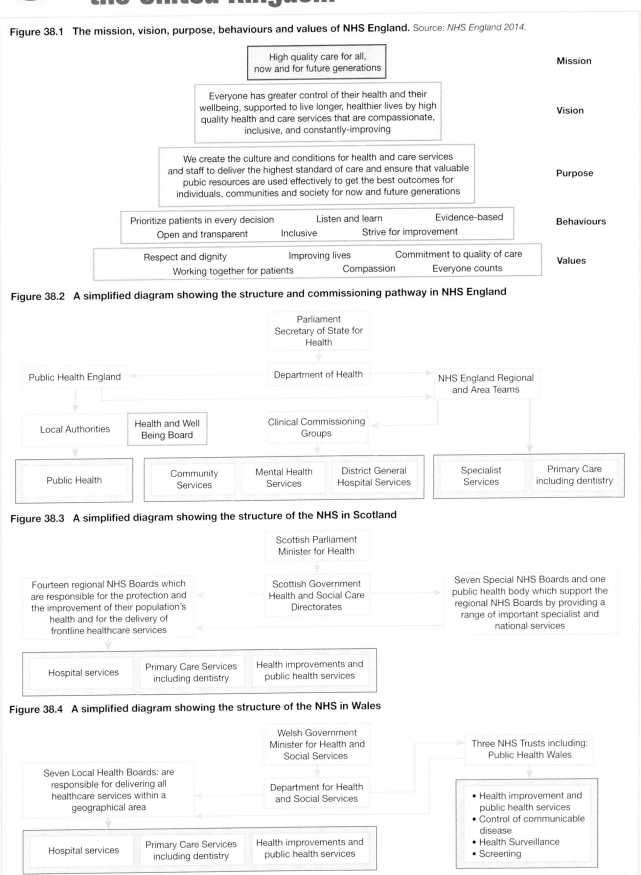

Figure 38.1 The mission, vision, purpose, behaviours and values of **NHS England.** Source: *NHS England 2014.*

| High quality care for all, now and for future generations | **Mission** |

Everyone has greater control of their health and their wellbeing, supported to live longer, healthier lives by high quality health and care services that are compassionate, inclusive, and constantly-improving — **Vision**

We create the culture and conditions for health and care services and staff to deliver the highest standard of care and ensure that valuable pubic resources are used effectively to get the best outcomes for individuals, communities and society for now and future generations — **Purpose**

Prioritize patients in every decision · Listen and learn · Evidence-based · Open and transparent · Inclusive · Strive for improvement — **Behaviours**

Respect and dignity · Improving lives · Commitment to quality of care · Working together for patients · Compassion · Everyone counts — **Values**

Figure 38.2 A simplified diagram showing the structure and commissioning pathway in NHS England

Parliament Secretary of State for Health

Public Health England · Department of Health · NHS England Regional and Area Teams

Local Authorities · Health and Well Being Board · Clinical Commissioning Groups

Public Health · Community Services · Mental Health Services · District General Hospital Services · Specialist Services · Primary Care including dentistry

Figure 38.3 A simplified diagram showing the structure of the NHS in Scotland

Scottish Parliament Minister for Health

Fourteen regional NHS Boards which are responsible for the protection and the improvement of their population's health and for the delivery of frontline healthcare services · Scottish Government Health and Social Care Directorates · Seven Special NHS Boards and one public health body which support the regional NHS Boards by providing a range of important specialist and national services

Hospital services · Primary Care Services including dentistry · Health improvements and public health services

Figure 38.4 A simplified diagram showing the structure of the NHS in Wales

Welsh Government Minister for Health and Social Services

Three NHS Trusts including: Public Health Wales

Seven Local Health Boards: are responsible for delivering all healthcare services within a geographical area · Department for Health and Social Services

- Health improvement and public health services
- Control of communicable disease
- Health Surveillance
- Screening

Hospital services · Primary Care Services including dentistry · Health improvements and public health services

Dental Public Health at a Glance, First Edition. Ivor G. Chestnutt.
© 2016 John Wiley & Sons, Ltd. Published 2016 by John Wiley & Sons, Ltd.

Primary dental care

General Dental Service (GDS)

The majority of dental care (85%) is provided in *primary care*, by general dental practitioners (GDPs). GDPs are independent practitioners who contract with the National Health Service (NHS) to provide an agreed volume of dental care. In England, practitioners contract with NHS England. In Wales and Scotland, dentists contract with local Health Boards. Traditionally GDS were provided by one or two dentists working from dental practices in the high street, often in buildings originally built for a purpose other than the provision of dental care. Increasingly, GDS services are being provided from multi-surgery, purpose-built premises and the contract may be held by a corporate body (company). In these circumstances the dentist, dental hygienist or dental therapist is often employed on a salaried basis.

Community/Salaried/Public Dental Services (CDS)

These services provide dental care for people whose social, medical and dental needs mean that they cannot be efficiently and effectively managed in the General Dental Service. Dental staff working in the CDS are salaried employees of the NHS. The CDS evolved from the School Dental Service in the mid-1970s. The degree to which it continues to act as a safety net service for high-need children in areas of social and economic deprivation varies across the United Kingdom. The CDS nowadays looks after elderly and housebound people and those with severe physical disabilities or mental illnesses.

In addition to the provision of care to high-need groups, the CDS provides staff who undertake local and national epidemiological studies of oral health. It is also responsible for the delivery of oral health promotion and education programmes and is intimately involved in national oral health improvement programmes such as Childsmile and Designed to Smile.

In Scotland the CDS is known as the Public Dental Service, while in England the term Salaried Dental Service is used.

Personal Dental Service (PDS)

This form of dental service allows for variation in the standard GDS and CDS commissioning arrangements and is used to procure specific types of service, such as domiciliary care or sedation services.

Secondary dental care

Hospital Dental Services (HDS)

Hospital dental services provide specialist dental care, either from general hospitals or from one of the dedicated dental hospitals. The most commonly provided services are oral and maxillofacial surgery and orthodontics. In dental hospitals the full range of dental specialist services is provided, including restorative dentistry, oral radiology and oral microbiology. Dental hospitals in conjunction with a local university also have responsibility for training the next generation of dental professionals.

Specialist dental care

It is possible for patients to access specialist dental care directly, usually outside the NHS on a private patient basis. Dentists who have undertaken additional specialist training and are registered on Specialist Lists held by the General Dental Council (GDC) may describe themselves as specialists and offer services directly to the public. Such practitioners often also take referrals from colleagues

in the GDS and provide treatments that are either too complex, for example oral surgery, or prohibitively expensive to provide under the GDS, for instance advanced endodontics or dental implants. Dental practitioners must not mislead patients into thinking that they possess additional specialist skills unless they are registered as a specialist with the GDC.

NHS and independent (private) dental care

The GDS, CDS and HDS provide care under the NHS. In addition, a substantial proportion of dental care is provided independently of the NHS. This enables patients to access routine care and care that is not provided under the NHS, such as cosmetic treatments or advanced restorative procedures. As independent contractors, GDPs may opt to provide all of their care independently, or to undertake mixed practice whereby they devote some of their time to providing care under an NHS contract and some outside the NHS. Care must be taken to ensure that patients are fully aware from the outset of the arrangements under which their care is being provided.

Patient involvement in dental care

In the past, healthcare professionals were seen as the possessors of wisdom and knowledge and largely instructed patients as to what they saw as being in the patients' best interests. Thankfully this attitude has changed and patients can now expect to be fully informed and involved in decisions about the options for their care. Dental professionals have a responsibility to ensure that their patients are fully appraised of all treatment options, the benefits, risks, consequences and costs of these options, before embarking on a course of treatment.

NHS England

NHS England (www.england.nhs.uk) was formed following the 2013 reorganization of the NHS in England. It is responsible for:
• Commissioning NHS services directly or via oversight of Clinical Commissioning Groups (CCGs), of which there are 211. NHS primary dental care is commissioned directly. NHS England is organized via 4 regional and 27 local area teams. Dentists contracting with the NHS work with staff from the local area teams to agree and monitor their contract.
• Improving patient experience.
• Patient involvement.
• Technology systems and data.
• Quality improvement and clinical leadership.

The mission, vision, purpose, behaviours and values of NHS England are shown in Figure 38.1. The position of NHS England within the overall structure of the NHS is illustrated in Figure 38.2. The structure of the NHS in Scotland and Wales is outlined in Figure 38.3 and 38.4.

Table 38.1 Definitions and examples of primary, secondary and tertiary care

Primary care – services that patients can access directly, e.g. General Dental Service, Community Dental Service, General Medical Service, pharmacists.
Secondary care – services that patients can access only on referral by a primary care practitioner, e.g. most hospital services, specialist NHS dental services.
Tertiary care – specialist services to which referrals are made by secondary care services, e.g. cleft lip and palate services.

③⑨ Paying for dental care

Table 39.1 Advantages and disadvantages of different systems of paying for dental services

Payment system	Fee per item	Capitation	Salary
Advantages	Provider paid for each item of treatment provided Provider incentivized to treat all existing disease	Commissioner can control costs more easily Allows both provider and commissioner to plan and budget more easily Advantageous to provider in low dental need patients	Beneficial when treating patients who require specialist care/whose treatment needs are more time consuming Allows commissioner to plan and budget more easily
Disadvantages	Risks overtreatment More difficult for commissioners to control costs	Risks undertreatment (supervised neglect) Potentially disadvantageous to provider in area of high dental need	Without effective management risks being inefficient

Table 39.2 Courses of treatment in the England and Wales NHS dental service (bands), their respective values (units of dental activity) and patient co-payments

Course of treatment	Treatment included	Units of dental activity[a]	Charge to non-exempt patients, NHS England (2015 prices)[b]
Band 1	Examination, scale and polish, radiographs and preventive treatments	1	£18.80
Band 2	Treatments in Band 1 plus restorations, root fillings and extractions	3	£51.30
Band 3	Treatments in Bands 1 and 2 plus crowns, bridges and dentures	12	£222.50
Urgent	Relief of pain/arrest of haemorrhage	1.2	As Band 1

[a]The average price paid per UDA to dentists by the NHS is £25.
[b]Patient charges in Wales are less that those levied in England.

Table 39.3 Public dental service entitlement and arrangements for patient co-payments in selected countries

Country	Population covered	Patient co-payment
Australia	Targeted groups only: adults on low incomes, those with chronic conditions or complex care needs; children and adolescents	Some dental services provided to eligible groups attract user charges, including school dental services; user charges vary regionally/locally
Canada	Targeted groups only: indigenous people, armed forces, refugees, local and provincial programmes (e.g. for individuals on low incomes)	Dental services provided to eligible user groups may attract user charges; these vary regionally/locally
England	Universal entitlement	Patients who are not exempt on the grounds of being < 18 years old, pregnant or nursing mother, receiving income support, pay one of three charges dependent on complexity of course of treatment
Finland	Universal entitlement	User charges are determined locally within limits set by the government; patients contribute 20% of costs on average
France	Universal entitlement under social health insurance	Social health insurance covers 70% of the costs of healthcare, including dental services; the remaining 30% is paid by the patient
Germany	Entitlement under social health insurance (covering about 88% of the population)	Some patient co-payment required – up to 50% in case of crowns. bridges and dentures
Netherlands	Universal entitlement to basic package of health services	Patients pay 25% of the cost of prostheses
New Zealand	Targeted groups only: individuals on low incomes or with complex care needs	Patients make a contribution to emergency dental care
Spain	Universal entitlement to acute dental care – more comprehensive treatment for children, pregnant women, disabled people and pensioners	Public dental services do not involve user charges
Sweden	Universal entitlement	Patients contribute to the cost of treatment on a sliding scale

Mechanisms of paying for dental care

There are three principal mechanisms of paying for dental care:
- **Fee per item** – where a charge is made for each item of treatment provided.
- **Capitation** – where the providing dentist receives a lump sum to provide care for a set number of patients.
- **Salary** – where the providing dentist is paid a salary to provide care. There are advantages and disadvantages to each of these payment systems (Table 39.1). They can be viewed from the perspective of both the provider of care (dental professional) and the commissioner of care (the NHS, insurance company or patient).

Current mechanisms of paying for dental care

National Health Service

The payment mechanism used varies across the United Kingdom. Over the last three decades several different payment systems have been employed in an attempt to ensure effective and efficient provision of NHS dental care. Traditionally NHS dentistry was based on a fee-per-item system of payment and this is still the main basis of payments to NHS GDS dentists in Scotland. The current arrangements in England and Wales are based on a system where dentists' output is measured in units of dental activity (UDA) and care is divided into three bands. This system, which was introduced in 2006, is widely recognized as flawed. The main drawback is the insensitivity to gradations of patient need. Under the UDA system a dentist gets paid the same fee for a patient who requires four restorations as for a patient who requires only one restoration (both qualify as Band 2 treatments). Dentists contract with NHS England or with the local Health Board in Wales (Chapter 38) to provide a specified number of UDAs on an annual basis. The clinical activity that falls within each of the three treatment bands, the UDAs that can be claimed and the patient co-payment are shown in Table 39.2.

Patient co-payments

To offset the costs of NHS dental care, patients are required to make a co-payment. In England and Wales this is one of three fees that relates to the treatment band provided in any course of treatment (Table 39.2). In Scotland, patients pay 80% of the cost of their treatment up to a maximum of £384 per course of treatment.

Those aged under 18 years, under 19 years and in full-time education, women who are pregnant or who have had a baby in the past 12 months and those in receipt of Income Support or income-related benefits are exempt from NHS patient charges.

At the time of writing, alternative ways of providing and paying for NHS dental care in England and Wales are being piloted (Chapter 43).

Dental professionals working in Hospital and Community Dental Services are paid a salary. Normally there is no patient co-charge for care provided in these settings, although in some circumstances charges are levied for prostheses.

Independent (private) dental care

Patients can either pay their dental provider directly on a fee-per-item basis, or join a dental insurance scheme, such as Denplan or BUPA. Typically for the latter the patient will pay a set monthly fee (which will vary according to their risk of future dental problems judged by their past treatment). This fee covers routine check-up examinations and basic care. Additional payments may be required if patients subsequently need more advanced restorative procedures such as crowns, bridges or implants.

Payment for dental services – international perspective

In the United Kingdom a very few individuals will have dental insurance provided by their employer. However, in the United States, employer-provided dental insurance is how most patients pay for their dental care. This means that those who are not employed or are employed in a low-grade job will not have any dental insurance. American children who are enrolled in the Medicaid programme are technically entitled to dental care – although the availability of willing dental care providers is a problem. While individual states are mandated to provide dental care for children, the provision of dental care for adults under the Medicaid programme is left to the state's discretion. Although most provide access to emergency dental care, less than half currently provide comprehensive dental coverage for poor and disadvantaged citizens.

In other countries, the provision of public dental services varies in relation to the proportion of the population covered and the degree to which patients must make a contribution towards the cost of their care. The position in some selected countries is illustrated in Table 39.3.

A blended dental contract

Given the pros and cons of different mechanisms of paying for public dental services, it is likely that an optimal system would involve a 'blended contract' whereby dentists receive a proportion of their income from capitation, allowances and a fee per item. This should be modelled to take into account the varying needs of the population served and the level of care that the commissioning body (that is, the government in the case of publicly funded services) wishes to provide. However, such a model is complex to devise and administer. Commissioning arrangements for dental care are discussed further in Chapter 43.

40 Barriers to accessing dental care

Figure 40.1 Self-reported dental attendance frequency by gender. Source: *Data from Health and Social Care Information Centre 2011.*

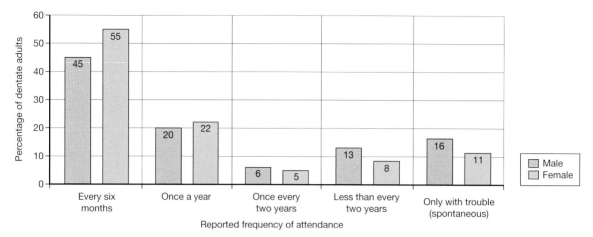

Figure 40.2 Potential barriers to accessing dental care

Patient related factors

- Perceived need
- Fatalistic attitude
- Lack of awareness
- Anxiety/fear
- Past dental experiences
- Disability - mental and/or physical
- Time availability - getting time off work
- Ethnic and cultural beliefs and practices

Dentist related factors

- Professional attitude
- Perceived competence of dentist by patients
- Availability of dentists with specialist skills

System related factors

- Cost
- Availability of NHS services
- Physical barriers - e.g. surgery accessible only via steps/stairs
- Rural and remote area issues
- Availability of transport

Table 40.1 Different types of need using dental attendance as an example

Need	Definition
Normative needs	Defined by experts, e.g. the frequency with which dental professionals recommend visiting a dentist
Felt needs	Those needs people say they have, e.g. a patient's description of how often they wish to visit a dentist
Expressed needs	Needs expressed by action, e.g. visiting a dentist
Comparative needs	Comparing one group of people with another, e.g. comparing dental attendance of different groups in relation to social and economic deprivation

Source: *Adapted from Bradshaw 1972.*

There are a number of barriers that may prevent a patient accessing dental care either at all, or as often as they need to or wish to.

Frequency of dental attendance

Guidance from the National Institute for Health and Care Excellence (NICE) recommends that recall intervals should be based on disease risk and vary between 3 and 24 months in adults. Data from the 2009 Adult Dental Health Survey (ADHS; (Figure 40.1) show that 50% of adults claimed to attend the dentist every six months, but 10% attend less often than every two years and a further 13% attend only when they have trouble with their teeth (symptomatic attendance). Successive ADHSs show that women attend the dentist more regularly than men. Just 2% of adults claimed never to have attended a dentist.

Barriers to dental care

Perceptions of need

In order that patients attend for care, they must feel or perceive the need to attend. Need can be viewed from different perspectives. It should be recognized that the perceptions of dental professionals and patients may differ when discussing the need for dental attendance. Definitions of need are shown in Table 40.1.

Patient attitudes as a barrier to care

Around a quarter of the population attend the dentist sporadically or only when provoked by a problem. This may reflect a lack of awareness of need, a fatalistic attitude or anxiety and fears about dental attendance.

Anxiety about dental attendance can be measured using the Modified Dental Anxiety Scale. This simple questionnaire asks potential patients to rate how worried they would be about attending the dentist and about the types of procedure that they might undergo during a dental appointment. In the 2009 ADHS, 30% of adults said that having a tooth drilled would make them very or extremely anxious and 28% reported similar levels of anxiety about having a local anaesthetic.

Costs as a barrier to care

The cost of dental care can be a barrier. This has been shown to prevent patients attending the dentist, to prevent patients having the treatment that they would like and to cause patients to delay or put off having treatment.

While the NHS dental system in the United Kingdom exempts patients who are receiving Income Support from co-payments (Chapter 39), in any means-tested system there are always those who just fail to qualify for welfare payments but for whom the cost of dental care may be a burden.

Dental professionals should make clear the costs of dental care at the commencement of treatment, and the General Dental Council requires that patients are given a written treatment plan with details of costs before treatment is carried out. The onus to be clear about costs lies with the dental team. Patients have reported that it may not be the actual cost that is the issue, but concerns over not knowing the cost and embarrassment about raising this issue when vulnerable in the dental chair that form the real barrier. Dentistry is one of the few areas of healthcare in the United Kingdom where patients have to pay at the point of delivery, and so patients may lack the confidence and skills to enquire about and negotiate costs, especially if paying directly out of their own pocket rather than via a dental insurance scheme.

Increasingly patients will desire treatments that are primarily for cosmetic purposes, such as tooth whitening or adult orthodontics, which may not be available via state-funded care. It is therefore important that information on costs and entitlement to treatment is made readily available to patients and prospective patients.

Availability of NHS care

As discussed in Chapter 38, dentists are independent contractors and can contract to provide as much or as little NHS care as they wish. Prior to 2006, NHS dental care was funded by a non-cash-limited budget and health authorities were obliged to contract with appropriately qualified and registered dentists. This is no longer the case and indeed, dentists can only opt to provide NHS care if they can negotiate a contract with NHS England or their local Health Board in Wales or Scotland.

In the early 2000s, lack of access to NHS care was an acute problem and pictures of patients queuing to register for NHS care were common in the media. However, by 2009, access to NHS dental care was less of a problem. The ADHS reported that 58% of adults said that they had tried to make an appointment with an NHS dentist in the previous three years. Of these, 92% successfully received and attended an appointment.

In the mid-2000s, an expansion in the number of dental students trained in the United Kingdom and an increase in the number of overseas dentists recruited to work in the NHS did much to ease problems in access to care.

Rural and remote communities

Access to dental care can be a problem in rural and remote communities. In addition to access to NHS dental services, issues such as distance to travel, lack of adequate public transport facilities and unwillingness on the part of young practitioners to work in rural and remote areas all contribute to the problem.

Access to care for patients with disabilities

Patients with mental and physical disabilities may experience difficulty in accessing care (Chapter 35).

Barriers interact in complex ways

Often issues over adequate access to dental care are not due to one single barrier but to a combination of factors that interact in complex ways and to greater or lesser degrees in any given patient (Figure 40.2).

41 Migration, race and ethnicity

Figure 41.1 The stages on a migrant's journey

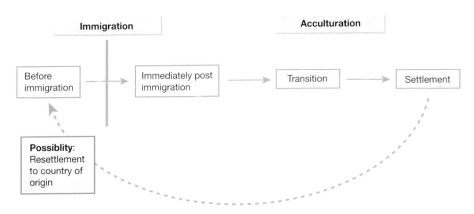

Table 41.1 Beliefs, traditions and cultural issues that may have impacts on dental care

Differences in habits, customs, beliefs, practices and other factors can have impacts on oral health-related behaviours and on the uptake and delivery of dental care. The following are issues with which members of the dental team should be familiar.

Factor	Issue	Examples
Health beliefs and understanding of disease	Different cultures have different health beliefs	Chinese people believe in the concept of yin and yang. This may influence their dietary choices, foods being balanced between yin (cold) and yang (hot). Remedies from traditional Chinese medicine may form part of their management of oral problems.
Gender issues and ideas of modesty	Religious protocol may dictate preferences when undergoing dental care	Modesty is important in all aspects of Muslim life and this extends to healthcare. Muslim women may prefer to be treated by female dentists.
Dietary restrictions	Avoidance of certain foods is important in many religions	Neither Jews nor Muslims eat pork. Certain dental materials, e.g. collagen sutures and periodontal chips, are porcine in origin. Patients should be made aware of this and an alternative agreed.
	Avoidance of alcohol is common in many religions	Strict observants will want to use an alcohol-free mouthwash. On occasion questions arise as to whether fluoride varnish is appropriate for the children of faiths that avoid alcohol (alcohol, present in trace amounts, acts as a solvent in fluoride varnish). Guidance from religious leaders suggests that this is not an issue. The alcohol is not consumed for pleasure and is not swallowed.
Fasting	Fasting is a common religious practice	During the holy month of Ramadan, Muslims fast from sun-up to sun-down. Patients may wish to avoid non-urgent dental treatment during this period and appointments should be scheduled accordingly.
Oral hygiene practices	Non-Western techniques of tooth cleaning may be preferred	Some patients, particularly older patients of Middle Eastern or African origin, may prefer to clean their teeth with a miswak – a fibrous root.
Different approaches to dental treatment	Approaches to dental treatment vary in different parts of the world	Dentistry in Eastern Europe (former Soviet bloc countries) often takes the form of 'heavy-duty' multiple fixed prostheses.
Tooth modification	Body modification and adornment have existed since the earliest times	Modification of the form and function of the dentition is still practised in many parts of the world and may be encountered when providing dental care. 'Dental grillz'/gold crowns in rappers are one current form of tooth adornment.
Language	Language-related issues	See Table 41.2.
Health literacy	Health literacy describes the ability to understand information related to health improvement and healthcare	Connected closely to language issues, unfamiliarity with Western dental care and practices can hinder understanding.
Torture	Asylum seekers may have been mistreated	Previous mistreatment involving the head and mouth as a form of punishment or torture should be borne in mind if treating a patient who has sought asylum.
Consent	For consent to treatment to be valid it needs to be informed	Where a dentist and patient do not share a common language, ensuring that the patient fully understands and agrees with proposed treatment can be a problem.

Dental Public Health at a Glance, First Edition. Ivor G. Chestnutt.
© 2016 John Wiley & Sons, Ltd. Published 2016 by John Wiley & Sons, Ltd.

The United Kingdom as a multicultural society

Data from the Office for National Statistics show that in 2013, of the 62.57 million usual residents in the United Kingdom, 1 in 8 (12.4% or 7.78 million) were born abroad. This compares to 1 in 11 (8.9%) in 2004. India was the most common non-UK country of birth – an estimated 734,000 usual residents in the United Kingdom were born in India. Polish is the most common non-British nationality – 726,000 usual residents in the United Kingdom have Polish nationality. It is therefore truly a multicultural society. This has implications for the organization and delivery of dental care.

Migration

A migrant is defined by the United Nations as:

a person who moves to a country other than that of his or her usual residence for a period of at least a year.

A number of different categories of migrants can be identified: migrant workers, students, asylum seekers and refugees, victims of trafficking and reunified family members.

Race and ethnicity

It is important to understand the difference between race and ethnicity.
- *Race is one of the major subdivisions of humankind, based largely on phenotypical differences between peoples.*
- *Ethnicity is a social construct that is based on common national or cultural traditions.*

There is very limited evidence that racial characteristics have any great impact on susceptibility to dental diseases. Some studies have suggested that some racial groups may be more susceptible to aggressive forms of periodontitis.

Of much greater significance is the impact of ethnic and cultural factors. Difference in habits, customs, beliefs and practices can have significant impacts on susceptibility to oral disease and to the uptake and acceptability of dental care, in a number of ways (Table 41.1).

Ethnicity and social and economic deprivation

The impact of social and economic factors on health is discussed in Chapter 19. It should always be remembered that minority communities frequently live in disadvantaged circumstances. In determining the impact of ethnic and cultural practices, the confounding effect of poverty needs to be carefully disentangled. Thus for example, do the higher rates of dental caries observed in black and minority ethnic (BME) children in England reflect underlying cultural practices, or is caries prevalence in these children no different from that in poor white children? Research studies are conflicting on the answer to this question.

Migration and health

Migrants' health can be influenced by factors at play during different stages of the immigration cycle (Figure 41.1). Typically, newly arrived immigrants are young and relatively healthy, but as they adapt to the lifestyle and practices in their adopted country (i.e. become acculturated), they more and more experience similar diseases to the indigenous population. Migrants tend to be more vulnerable to diabetes, certain communicable diseases, maternal and child health problems, occupational health hazards and poor mental health. Obesity is increasingly recognized as a problem when migrants move from a low-income to a developed country.

Access to healthcare

Access to healthcare can be a particular problem for migrants. Language issues are often a barrier and steps to overcome these are shown in Table 41.2. General health literacy, social exclusion and discrimination (both obvious and concealed) are further barriers.

Irregular (illegal) immigrants, who do not comply with entry, exit, visa and work permit requirements, are particularly likely to experience difficulty in accessing health services.

Migrant clinicians and health workers

The National Health Service has for many years relied on healthcare professionals trained overseas to meet its workforce requirements. In addition, a growing number of dependent elderly people in nursing and care homes often rely on low-skilled migrant workers to provide basic care.

Overseas trained dentists

Dentists who have qualified at a dental school in the European Union are entitled to work in the United Kingdom under freedom of movement regulations. The European Directive on the Recognition of Professional Qualifications for Dentists enables European Economic Area (EEA) nationals who qualified at a dental school in the EEA to practise anywhere in the EEA without the need to undertake further education or training. Recent years have seen many dentists of Eastern European nationality come to work in the United Kingdom. This was particularly encouraged in the early 2000s by the NHS as a means of addressing the then acute problem of access to NHS dentistry. Dentists who qualify outside the EEA must pass the Overseas Registration Examination (ORE), administered by the General Dental Council, before they can undertake independent practice in the United Kingdom.

Differences in competencies acquired during undergraduate training and unfamiliarity with NHS Dental Regulations are potential problems for dentists coming to work in the United Kingdom. NHS Commissioners have been proactive in organizing additional skills training for practitioners in this position.

Cultural competence

In an increasingly diverse society, it is important that both healthcare organizations and healthcare professionals are *culturally competent*. This means that they need to be aware of the types of issues addressed in this chapter.

Table 41.2 Options to manage an encounter when clinician and patient do not share a common language

Method of translation	Notes
Face-to face translation by a friend or relative	The most common, but least satisfactory method; can be difficult to ensure that the dentist is hearing the patient's view and not the relative's view
Face-to face translation by a professional translator	The preferred option; not always available; expensive; needs arranging in advance; may not be available in an emergency situation
Use of a professional telephone translation service	Lacks the face-to face element – difficult when undertaking treatment
Use of bilingual cards and photographs	Can be of some help, particularly if the parties share a little of a common language – not possible to have to hand all of the many languages that could possibly be encountered

Skill mix in dentistry

Table 42.1 Total number of people on the Dentists Register and the Dental Care Professionals Register at the end of 2013, by gender

		Male	Female
Dentist	41,007 (39%)	22,126 (54%)	18,880 (46%)
Dental care professional (DCP)	64,939 (61%)	5,770 (9%)	59,169 (91%)
Total	**105,946**	**27,896**	**78,049**

Source: *Data from General Data Council 2014.*

Table 42.2 Total number of titles on the Dentists Register and the Dental Care Professionals Register at the end of 2013, by gender

Registration type	Number	Percentage of all registrants
Dentist	41,007	37.4
Clinical dental technician	304	0.3
Dental hygienist	6,548	6.0
Dental nurse	52,552	48.0
Dental technician	6,292	5.7
Dental therapist	2,455	2.2
Orthodontic therapist	407	0.4
Total	**109,565**	**100**

N.B. *Number of titles is greater than the number of people as an individual may be registered in more than one registration type.*
Source: *Data from General Data Council 2014.*

Table 42.3 Scope of practice of dental therapists in the UK

Dental therapists are registered dental professionals who provide certain items of dental treatment direct to patients or under prescription from a dentist.

If trained, competent and appropriately indemnified, dental therapists can:
• Obtain a detailed dental history from patients and evaluate their medical history.
• Carry out a clinical examination within their competence.
• Complete periodontal examination and charting and use indices to screen and monitor periodontal disease.
• Diagnose and devise a treatment plan within their competence.
• Prescribe radiographs.
• Take, process and interpret various film views used in general dental practice.
• Plan the delivery of care for patients.
• Give appropriate patient advice.
• Provide preventive oral care to patients and liaise with dentists over the treatment of caries, periodontal disease and tooth wear.
• Undertake supragingival and subgingival scaling and root surface debridement using manual and powered instruments.
• Use appropriate antimicrobial therapy to manage plaque-related diseases.
• Adjust restored surfaces in relation to periodontal treatment.
• Apply topical treatments and fissure sealants.
• Give patients advice on how to stop smoking.
• Take intra- and extraoral photographs.
• Give infiltration and inferior dental block analgesia.
• Place temporary dressings and re-cement crowns with temporary cement.
• Place rubber dam.
• Take impressions.
• Take care of implants and provide treatment for peri-implant tissues.
• Carry out direct restorations on primary and secondary teeth.
• Carry out pulpotomies on primary teeth.
• Extract primary teeth.
• Place pre-formed crowns on primary teeth.
• Identify anatomical features, recognize abnormalities and interpret common pathology.
• Carry out oral cancer screening.
• If necessary, refer patients to other healthcare professionals.
• Keep full, accurate and contemporaneous patient records.
• If working on prescription, vary the detail but not the direction of the prescription according to patient needs. For example, the number of surfaces to be restored or other material to be used.

Additional skills that dental therapists could develop include:
• Carrying out tooth whitening to the prescription of a dentist.
• Administering inhalation sedation.
• Removing sutures after the wound has been checked by a dentist.
All other skills are reserved to orthodontic therapists, dental technicians, clinical dental technicians or dentists.

Source: *Data from General Data Council 2013.*

Dental Public Health at a Glance, First Edition. Ivor G. Chestnutt.
© 2016 John Wiley & Sons, Ltd. Published 2016 by John Wiley & Sons, Ltd.

The concept of skill mix

The tasks required to provide comprehensive healthcare are not of equal complexity. As both the number of staff and the amount of finance in any healthcare system are finite, the delivery of healthcare can be made more efficient by the use of a mix of staff, trained to different levels. This allows the most highly trained staff to delegate aspects of care to other professionals. This concept is known as **skill mix**. It has been widely adopted in medicine and many procedures that would previously have been conducted by a medical practitioner are now delegated to a nurse. Skill mix in dentistry currently lags behind that in medicine.

Skill Mix in Dentistry

The idea of dental care professionals (previously termed auxiliaries) has been in existence for 100 years and in 1916, the School Dental Service in the United Kingdom employed dental dressers (the equivalent of dental therapists). These workers were phased out in the early 1920s following the passing of the Dentists Act 1921. The first dental hygienists in the United Kingdom were trained by the military in 1943, with civilian schools of dental hygiene being established in the 1950s. Training of dental therapists began formally in the 1960s in London. Until the early 2000s, dental therapists were restricted to working in Hospital and Community Dental Services, but changed legislation means that dental therapists can now work in general dental practice.

The concept of dental care, delivered by a multiskilled team, was given prominence by a report from the Nuffield Foundation in 1993 and subsequently endorsed by a General Dental Council (GDC) sponsored review of the use of dental auxiliaries in 1998. The model of a primary care dental team, led by a dentist who diagnoses, prescribes and delegates routine clinical care to a team of support professionals (dental nurses, hygienists, therapists and technicians), is now accepted in the United Kingdom.

All dentists and dental care professionals (DCPs) are required to register with the GDC. The number of individuals registered and the range of DCPs recognized by the GDC are shown in Tables 42.1 and 42.2.

In the past two decades the range of tasks that DCPs can train to undertake has expanded markedly. In 2013, the GDC granted *direct access* to some categories of DCP. This means that patients can see dental hygienists and therapists without first having seen a dentist or without the need for a prescription, although the precise details of how this will work and the impact that this will have on the delivery of dental care are still being established.

Tasks that can be undertaken by dental care professionals

The list of competencies expected of all dental professionals is set out in guidance from the GDC entitled *Preparing for Practice– Dental Team Learning, Outcomes for Registration* (www.gdc-uk.org). As for dentists, the proficiencies required of DCPs are described in four domains:

- Clinical
- Communication
- Professionalism
- Management and leadership.

The scope of practice of individual registrant groups is also defined by the GDC and sets out the areas of dental practice that a given professional group could be expected and trained to perform. These are set out in detail for dentists and for each DCP group in a GDC publication, *Scope of Practice 2013*. The scope of practice for dental therapists is shown in Table 42.3.

Dentists should be aware of the range of skills and duties that fall within the remit of each DCP group and delegate care accordingly. Like dentists, DCPs have a duty to undertake life-long learning and to make an annual return to the GDC to enable their ongoing registration (Chapter 44). It is expected that DCPs will have the opportunity to develop and enhance their skills in the course of a career in practice.

Skill mix – an international perspective

Dental therapists

The first formal training programme for dental therapists was established in New Zealand in 1923. with two further schools opened in the 1950s. It was largely the success of the New Zealand model that encouraged the establishment of a training programme in London in the 1960s. Despite the long history of dental therapists treating children in New Zealand and the United Kingdom, the concept of dental therapists has not been widely adopted around the world. Often vested interests and the strength of national dental associations have been set against the development of this class of dental professional. At present, vigorous debate continues in the United States as to the merits of employing dental therapists, despite many thousands of uninsured high-need children in that country who do not have access to routine dental care.

Dental hygienists

Dental hygienists, with their more restricted remit, have seen much wider acceptance by the dental profession across the world. Dental hygienists are widely employed in Scandinavian countries and in the United States. However, they are much less common in southern European countries and are not used in Austria, Belgium, France, Greece or Luxembourg.

Dental nurses

While the concept of four-handed dentistry is firmly established in the United Kingdom and many other countries, the use of dental nurses or dental assistants is not universal. Direct chairside assistants are relatively uncommon in Luxembourg and France.

Clinical dental technicians

As well as being registered in the United Kingdom, clinical dental technicians are found in Denmark and France, where they can provide removable dental prostheses directly to patients.

43 A vision for the future delivery of dental care

Figure 43.1 Proposed patient pathway as described in the 2009 Independent review of NHS Denistry - "the Steele Review". Source: *Steele et al. 2009. Available through the Open Government Licence for public sector information. http://www.nationalarchives.gov.uk/doc/open-government-licence/version/3/*

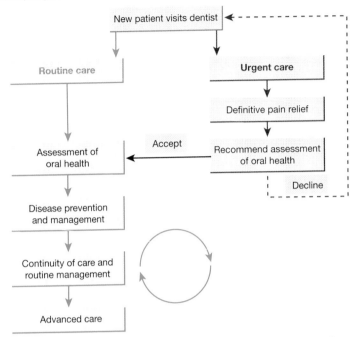

Figure 43.2 The preventive care pathway being tested as the model for reorientating NHS dental care. Source: *Department of Health 2015. Available through the Open Government Licence for public sector information. http://www.nationalarchives.gov.uk/doc/open-government-licence/version/3/*

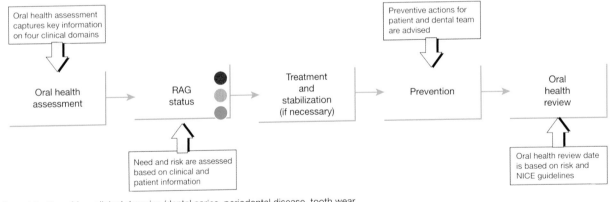

A combination of four clinical domains (dental caries, periodontal disease, tooth wear and soft tissue pathology) combined with patient factors (e.g. level of plaque control) are used to produce a RAG status (red, amber, green) - indicating disease risk.

The challenges ahead

The main challenges facing the delivery of dental care in the United Kingdom in the future are summarized in Box 43.1.

NHS dentistry 1948 to present

When the NHS was established in 1948, oral health in the United Kingdom was extremely poor. However, universal access to dentistry generated by the NHS in the mid-twentieth century meant that patients could be relieved of grossly decayed teeth and provided with complete or partial dentures, which adequately restored form and function, met patients' needs and were a vast improvement in standards at the time. Such was the demand for dental care that in 1952, the concept of dental care free for all at the point of delivery was abandoned, as it became obvious that the state could not afford to pay for all of the dental care the public wished to consume. Means-tested patient charges (co-payments) were introduced. For the remainder of the twentieth century, under a fee-per-item method of payment, the efforts of NHS dentists did much to improve the oral health of the nation (Chapter 9).

Since the 1960s, various reviews and investigations into NHS dentistry have resulted in changes to how dentists are remunerated. Many of these changes were designed to address the pros and cons of remunerating dentists using fee-per-item versus capitation (Chapter 39). The most significant changes occurred in 1990 and 2006. The last major change in England and Wales happened in 2006 and introduced the concept of units of dental activity and payment bands. It also for the first time put a limit on the total money available for NHS dentistry each year.

Within a short period of time it was recognized that the 2006 contract reforms were failing to meet the desired objectives – simplifying the payment system and increasing access to NHS dentistry. The main issue was that transition from a fee-per-item system with over 400 items to a system with effectively three items was not working.

NHS dentistry in the future

The Department of Health in England commissioned an independent review of NHS dentistry in 2009. Led by Professor Jimmy

Steele, this review proposed a future model of NHS dentistry as shown in Figure 43.1. This suggests the availability of urgent care for everyone when required and the opportunity to enter continuing care. The model suggested a care pathway in which a patient's oral health and risk of future disease are assessed. The focus of care should be on prevention, tailored to the patient's individual needs. Advanced aspects of care would only be provided when there is a stable oral environment, the patient's disease risks are under control and the patient is in a continuing care relationship with the dentist/dental team.

The expectation is that adult patients would attend at intervals of between 3 and 24 months, as recommended by NICE Guidelines on Dental Recall. The 'Steele Review', as this report has become known, emphasized that the priority for *NHS dental care was to refocus from a service designed to provide restorative care to one that focused on prevention.*

NHS dental pilots

In the period since the publication of the Steele Review, the Department of Health in England and the Welsh Government have conducted 'contract reform pilots'. The government is keen to point out that these pilots are about not only how to pay for dental services under the NHS, but also reshaping how care is delivered in line with the ethos of more prevention and less restoration. The concepts underling the contracts being piloted were registration of patients with a dentist, capitation as a means of paying the dentist and quality in terms of what is delivered.

In January 2015, the Department of Health announced its intention to move from pilots to testing **prototypes** of a new NHS dental contract. The purpose of these prototypes is to test possible new systems of delivering and paying for NHS dental care; in the pilots only parts of any new system were tested. As well as capitation, the prototypes will include an element of payment for activity (i.e. payment related to certain clinical procedures). The combination of capitation and activity is known as a **blended contract**.

The 2015 prototype contracts will consist of:
- A clinical pathway (Figure 43.2).
- A set of clinical measures (Dental Quality and Outcomes Framework or DQOF), based around the preventive activities set out in *Delivering Better Oral Health* and the NICE guidance on recall intervals.
- Remuneration better aligned with access and clinical outcomes (a **blend** of quality, capitation and activity).

Given the deficiencies of the 2006 reforms, the Department of Health is keen to emphasize that the new system of care being devised is one of evolution, not revolution. As a result, it intends to test any new system thoroughly. It is currently (November 2015) envisaged that any new system will not form the majority contract approach until 2018–19 at the earliest.

Box 43.1 Factors with the potential to influence the future delivery of dental care in the UK

- Increasing population (absolute numbers)
- Ageing population
- Increased tooth retention into old age
- Changed attitudes to oral health
- Public less willing to accept extractions
- Ever-rising expectations for good dental appearance
- Need to address inequalities in oral health
- Ever-improving dental technology, which means teeth can be restored that previously would have been extracted
- Advances in restorative dental materials
- Increased demand for cosmetic dental care
- Limited resources to fund NHS dentistry
- Difficulty in workforce planning – the numbers of dental students being trained in the United Kingdom over the past three decades has been reduced, expanded and reduced again
- Global mobility and European employment legislation have resulted in a much greater number of overseas dentists working in the United Kingdom
- The enactment of *direct access* powers for dental hygienists and therapists means that greater use of skill mix is likely than has previously been the case

---

Independent dental practice

The independent contractor status of general dental practitioners (Chapter 39) means that dentists can deliver care on a private basis. Given that funds available for providing NHS dental care are finite, people who want to have more advanced forms of care such as implants or cosmetic dental procedures will have to seek these outside the NHS. However, the NHS reforms make clear that patients will be able to choose such treatments alongside NHS care should they so desire.

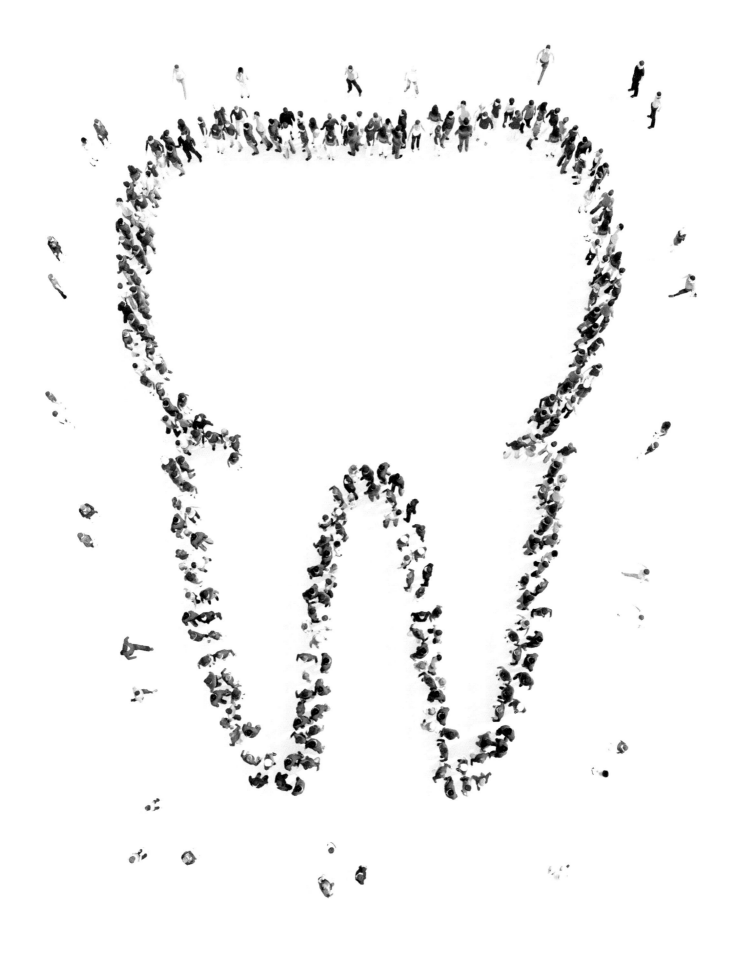

Quality assurance of dental care

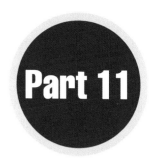

Part 11

Chapters

44 Quality dental care

Figure 44.1 The components of quality healthcare

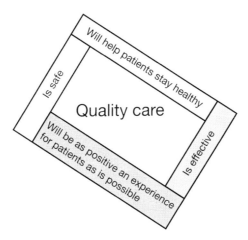

Quality care

Is safe

Will help patients stay healthy

Will be as positive an experience for patients as is possible

Is effective

Table 44.1 Possible consequences of failing to provide quality dental care

A patient may:

- Fail to return for further appointments.
- Tell their family and friends that they are dissatisfied with your care and do not recommend your practice. There have been examples of patients posting adverse comments on the internet or social media when dissatisfied with their dental care.
- Complain to the dental practice.
- Complain to the NHS Commissioners, to their insurance provider or to the General Dental Council.
- Seek legal redress (sue the dentist or other member of the dental team).

Table 44.3 Examples of risks that need to be managed in dental practice

- Health and safety
  - Slips, trips and falls
  - Cross-infection control
  - Radiation protection
  - Hazardous substances (Committee on Substances Hazardous to Health [COSHH] regulations)
  - Fire evacuation
- Management of medical emergencies
- Patient identification
- Medical records
- Data protection
- Complaints

Table 44.2 Continuing Professional Development (CPD) – requirements as set out by the General Dental Council (2013)

Minimum CPD hours	
Dentists 250 hours of CPD every 5 years, of which 75 hours must be *verifiable*	*Dental care professionals* 150 hours of CPD every 5 years, of which 75 hours must be *verifiable*

Verifiable CPD	**Non-verifiable CPD**
Verifiable CPD is an activity for which there is documentary evidence of participation. Such activity should have: • concise educational aims and objectives • clear anticipated outcomes • quality controls.	This is educational activity that does not necessarily have evidence of participation.

CDP activity	**Highly recommended CPD topics**
The following activities can contribute to CPD: • Courses and lectures • Training days • Peer review • Clinical audit • Reading journals • Attending conferences • E-learning activity	• Medical Emergencies – at least 10 hours in every CPD cycle, at least 2 hours per year • Disinfection and decontamination – at least 5 hours in every CPD cycle • Radiography and radiation protection – at least 5 hours in every CPD cycle Other recommended topics: • Legal and ethical issues • Complaints handling • Early detection of oral cancer

---

Dental Public Health at a Glance, First Edition. Ivor G. Chestnutt.

Quality in healthcare

Quality equates to a degree or standard of excellence. Patients quite rightly expect care to be of a certain standard and to maximize their health. There are three components to high-quality care: *clinical effectiveness*, *safety* and *patient experience* (Figure 44.1).

These concepts encompass the six dimensions of healthcare quality defined by Maxell in 1984 as:

- Access to services
- Relevance to need (for the whole community)
- Effectiveness (for individual patients)
- Equity (fairness)
- Social acceptability
- Efficiency and economy.

In an era when patients increasingly have to pay directly for dental care and when dental practitioners are in effect running a business, as in other walks of life patients expect a quality service. Recent high-profile failures in the provision of healthcare such as that observed at the Mid-Staffordshire NHS Foundation Trust, where serious deficiencies in the commissioning, organization and delivery of healthcare were ignored, have heightened the focus on providing quality healthcare and ensuring that mechanisms are in place to monitor the provision of care.

The possible consequences of failing to provide quality dental care are shown in Table 44.1.

Clinical governance

Clinical governance is a framework that is designed to ensure that the quality of care patients receive is of a high standard. It is, as the current jargon goes, **about ensuring that patients get the right care at the right time from the right person and that it happens right first time**. The formal definition of clinical governance is:

A framework through which NHS organisations are accountable for continuously improving the quality of their services and safeguarding high standards of care by creating an environment in which excellence in clinical care will flourish. (Scally and Donaldson 1998)

Clinical governance has the following main components:

1 Clinical audit – see Chapter 45.

2 Clinical effectiveness and evidence-based dentistry – see Chapter 18.

3 Research and development – healthcare providers are encouraged to participate in research to inform the development of evidence for best practice.

4 Continuing professional development (CPD) – it is expected that all healthcare professionals will take steps to keep themselves up to date throughout their practising careers. This is monitored by the General Dental Council (GDC) and all registered dental professionals must make an annual return to confirm that they are compliant with the minimum expectations. The GDC determines a minimum number of hours that must be committed to CPD over a five-year period and has also identified key topics that should be covered (Table 44.2).

5 Risk management – the practice of dentistry and the dental environment pose risks to patients, staff and visitors. Dental professionals have a duty to manage such risks and to minimize harm to patients by:

- Identifying what can and does go wrong in the delivery of dental care.
- Understanding the factors that influence this.
- Learning lessons from any adverse events.
- Ensuring that action is taken to prevent recurrence.
- Putting systems in place to reduce risk.

The major risks that need to be managed in a dental practice are shown in Table 44.3.

6 Effective management of poorly performing staff – dentists have a responsibility to ensure that staff working under their supervision are effectively managed and supported. Dental staff may underperform for many reasons, including:

- Professional isolation
- Workload problems
- Lack of continuing professional development (CPD)
- Low morale
- Poor health related to physical or mental problems, alcohol or stress
- Family/other problems outside work.

Dental professionals have an obligation to take action if they suspect that the performance of a colleague or member of staff is such that it may jeopardise the health or welfare of patients or other members of the team. Arrangements should be in place for staff to raise concerns in a confidential manner (*whistle-blowing; i.e. making a disclosure in the public interest*) without fear of retribution.

Formal bodies such as the National Patient Safety Agency (NPSA) aim to reduce risks to patients receiving NHS care. NPSA leads on national initiatives to improve patient safety.

7 Involvement of patients – it is crucial to a quality dental service that patients' views and wishes are taken into account. This may be facilitated by the Patient Advice and Liaison Service (PALS), which offers confidential advice and support on healthcare-related matters. A similar function is fulfilled by the Community Health Councils in Wales and by the Scottish Health Council.

45 Clinical audit

Figure 45.1   The clinical audit cycle

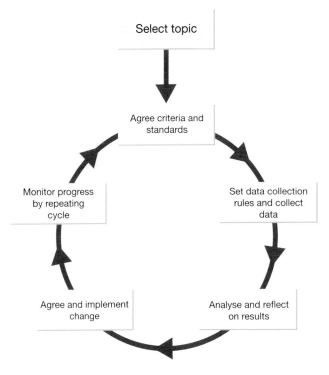

Select topic

Agree criteria and standards

Set data collection rules and collect data

Analyse and reflect on results

Agree and implement change

Monitor progress by repeating cycle

Table 45.1 Reasons for undertaking clinical audit

- Improved care of patients
- Enhanced professionalism of staff
- Efficient use of resources
- Aid to administration of dental practice
- Aid to continuing education
- Accountability to those outside the profession
- Requirement of employing organizations and often a condition of employment

Table 45.2 The features of a good clinical audit project

- Effective at improving care
- Not too complicated
- Has a clear purpose
- Assists staff
- Not used as a means of discipline
- Confidential

Table 45.3 Practical issues that may limit the implementation of clinical audit

- Often audits do not complete the loop due to participant fatigue
- Clinical audit may be seen as a threat or implied criticism
- Viewed as time consuming
- May choose topics that are not clinically important or significant
- There is an 'opportunity cost' in doing the audit – time spent on audit activities cannot be spent doing something else

Dental Public Health at a Glance, First Edition. Ivor G. Chestnutt.
© 2016 John Wiley & Sons, Ltd. Published 2016 by John Wiley & Sons, Ltd.

Clinical audit

Clinical audit is central to ensuring that quality dental care is being delivered. Clinical audit can be defined as follows:

Clinical audit is the process of reviewing the delivery of healthcare to identify deficiencies so that they may be remedied.

Clinical audit is a cyclical process in which current care is compared with a standard and changes implemented if the standard is not being achieved (Figure 45.1). The rationale and benefits of clinical audit are shown in Table 45.1.

The clinical audit cycle

Clinical audit involves the following steps.

1 Deciding on the topic for audit

The topic chosen for audit should relate to a clinically important aspect of care or significant event. Subjects for audit may be identified by the observations of staff or arise from patient comments or complaints. Clinical guidelines may also highlight suitable topics for audit.

2 Agree criteria and standards

A **criterion** is a specific statement of what should be happening.

A **standard** is a minimum level of acceptable performance.

For some topics, criteria and standards are defined by clinical guidelines, for instance the standards produced by the Royal College of Radiologists on the quality of radiographs, or by the National Institute for Health and Care Excellence (NICE) on the frequency of dental recall intervals. For other topics there are no national guidelines and it is up to the team conducting the audit to agree their own acceptable criteria and standards, as in the following examples:

Criterion	Standard
All patients should have a completed, up-to-date medical history before treatment commences	Minimum 100%
All patients should be seen within 15 minutes of their appointment time	Minimum 75%

Here it is clear that the standard for up-to-date medical histories should be 100%, but in the case of keeping patients waiting beyond their appointed treatment time, the standard would be a matter for local decision making.

3 Data collection

The data required for the audit may already be available from patients' records. Electronic patient record systems have greatly facilitated the retrieval of information on all patients who underwent a particular procedure and avoids the lengthy process of data retrieval from paper-based records.

The information necessary to conduct an audit may need to be collected prospectively via a data collection chart or questionnaire. It is important that the data collection process is kept as simple as possible and that the audit is restricted to a clearly defined aspect of practice. Often a simple tally chart collected by pen and paper is sufficient for the purposes of clinical audit.

The time over which the data is collected should be as short as is commensurate with collecting sufficient information to get a picture of what is happening. For example, the agreement may be to collect information on the next 100 consecutively attending patients. Alternatively, data could be collected for all patients over a two-week period. Unlike in research studies, there is no need for a 'power calculation' to determine the required numbers.

4 Data analysis and reflection on results

Data analysis is usually restricted to simple counts and frequency analysis. There is no need for the application of statistical tests or calculation of probability values in clinical audit. The purpose of the analysis is to determine whether current practice meets the minimum standard agreed.

5 Agree and implement change

If the minimum standard is not being met, then it is necessary to agree and implement change to achieve the standard. Managing change is one of the greatest challenges that managers face. If changes are required, then there needs to be agreement on what changes are necessary, who is going to be responsible for making the changes, when this will occur and how. Staff can be reluctant to change and it is important that they understand the reason for change and are provided with the necessary skills and resources to make change possible.

6 Monitor progress by repeating the cycle

What makes clinical audit a *cyclical process* is the necessity to repeat the audit some time after the changes have been implemented to see whether they have had the desired effect and the minimum standard is now being achieved.

Features of a good clinical audit project

The features of a good clinical audit project are described in Table 45.2.

Practical aspects of clinical audit

The practical aspects that can limit the implementation of clinical audit are shown in Table 45.3.

Donabedian's triad

Donabedian described three elements of approaching healthcare quality. Clinical audits can be considered under these three headings:

- *Structure* – looks at amount and nature of staff, and facilities.
- *Process* – looks at what is actually done to patients.
- *Outcome* – looks at the results of treatment.

Peer review

Peer review is a quality assurance mechanism that operates alongside clinical audit. Peer review is less structured and less formal than clinical audit. In peer review, practitioners gather to discuss a clinical topic of mutual interest, often sharing details of clinical cases or problems. The theory is that by sharing ideas, solutions and standards will emerge by mutual consensus and participants will learn from each other.

The difference between clinical audit and research

It is very important to appreciate the difference between clinical audit and clinical research.

- *Clinical research* is about extending the body of knowledge of best practice.
- *Clinical audit* is about measuring whether best practice is being applied.

46 Regulatory bodies and patient complaints

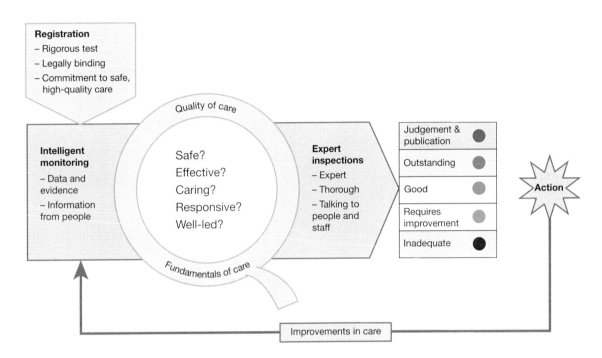

Figure 46.1 Care Quality Commission's Operating model. Source: *Care Quality Commission 2014. Available under the Open Government Licence http://www.nationalarchives.gov.uk/doc/open-government-licence/version/2/*

Table 46.1 The functions of the General Dental Council

Maintain the Dental Register
The GDC maintains registers of all dental professionals. This comprises registers of dentists and dental care professionals. The GDC also maintains a list of 13 dental specialties, which sets out who has undertaken additional training and is qualified as a Specialist. The registers are available online (www.gdc.org) and are searchable by anyone.
Investigate concerns and complaints about dental professionals
Through a *Fitness to Practice Committee*, the GDC investigates concerns about dental professionals. These may be on the grounds of *health; conduct* including convictions and cautions; and *performance*. Investigation can lead to a number of outcomes for the dental professional concerned: • Being struck off the Dental Register so that they can no longer practise as a dental professional • Suspension for a set period of time • Being set conditions that restrict their practice • A reprimand (a statement of disapproval) • A finding of no case to answer
Set and maintain educational standards
The GDC has defined the educational requirements for educational courses that qualify dentists and dental care professionals for entry to the Dental Register or Specialists Lists. The GDC undertakes a series of inspections of dental schools and educational providers to ensure that the courses provided and assessment of students undertaking these courses are of a minimum standard.
Continuing professional development
The GDC sets the requirements and maintains the record of continuing professional development for all dental professionals.
Overseas Registration Examination (ORE)
This examination, designed for dentists who have qualified outside the European Economic Area (EEA), is overseen by the GDC and successful completion allows dentists to practise unsupervised in the UK.
Provision of information to patients
The GDC occasionally issues information for the public on topics of current interest, e.g. tooth whitening or travelling abroad to have dental treatment.

Dental Public Health at a Glance, First Edition. Ivor G. Chestnutt.
© 2016 John Wiley & Sons, Ltd. Published 2016 by John Wiley & Sons, Ltd.

The regulation of dentistry

Dentistry is a profession regulated by statute, Section 38 of the Dentists Act 1984. It is therefore illegal for an individual to practise dentistry if they are not appropriately qualified and registered with the General Dental Council. The illegal practice of dentistry can lead to a criminal conviction and fine.

General Dental Council

The General Dental Council is responsible for the regulation of the dental profession in the United Kingdom. Its functions are set out by Parliament, although it operates independently of both the government and the NHS. All dental professionals (Chapter 42), irrespective of which sphere of dentistry they practise in, must be registered with the GDC and pay an annual fee to remain on the register.

The Council is made up of *six appointed registrants* and *six appointed lay members*. It is the responsibility of the Council to ensure that the core responsibility of protecting patients is fulfilled.

The GDC describes its main functions as *protecting patients* and *regulating the dental profession*. This is achieved as set out in Table 46.1.

The nine professional principles

The GDC has set out nine principles to which all registrants and dental students must adhere:

1 Put patients' interests first.
2 Communicate effectively with patients.
3 Obtain valid consent.
4 Maintain and protect patients' information.
5 Have a clear and effective complaints procedure.
6 Work with colleagues in a way that is in patients' best interests.
7 Maintain, develop and work within your professional knowledge and skills.
8 Raise concerns if patients are at risk.
9 Make sure your personal behaviour maintains patients' confidence in you and the dental profession.

These standards are described in detail in a GDC publication, *Standards for the Dental Team* (www.gdc.org.uk). Failure to adhere to these standards can result in referral to the GDC and investigation under its 'fitness to practise' procedures.

The Care Quality Commission (CQC)

The Care Quality Commission (CQC) is the independent regulator of health and social care in England. All dental providers in England must register with the CQC. Its purpose is to ensure that health and social care services provide people with safe, effective, compassionate, high-quality care and to encourage care services to improve. The CQC's operating model is shown in Figure 46.1.

The role of the CQC is to inspect and regulate services to make sure that they meet fundamental standards of quality and safety. It publishes the results of inspections and for some services (although not currently in dentistry) the CQC includes performance ratings to help people choose care. Dentists must pay an annual fee to remain registered with the CQC.

Following inspection of a dental practice, the CQC will report on compliance in the following areas:
• Treating people with respect and involving them in their care.
• Providing care, treatment and support that meet people's needs.
• Caring for people safely and protecting them from harm.
• Staffing.
• Quality and suitability of management.

Failure to meet the required standard may result in the issue of an enforcement notice.

Health Inspectorate Wales performs a similar function to the CGC in Wales. In Scotland dental practices are subject to inspection by Health Boards on a three-year cycle, and plans are also afoot for private dental practices to be inspected by **Healthcare Improvement Scotland (HIS).**

Patient complaints

The most common causes of complaint in dental practice are failure in communication, disputes over monetary charges and failure of clinical treatment.

Effective and efficient management of patients' concerns and complaints is important, as resolution at an early stage may prevent the scenarios outlined in Table 44.1. It is always preferable that a patient's complaint or concern be resolved informally. However, if the patient wishes to complain formally, then the options available depend on whether their treatment was carried out under the National Health Service or Independently.

The NHS complaints process

This has two stages:
• *Stage 1 – Local resolution.* Here the patient makes a formal complaint to the dentist or to the commissioner of the service. If the patient remains unsatisfied with the solution offered, then Stage 2 may be involved.
• *Stage 2 – Complaint to the Parliamentary and Health Service Ombudsman.* This stage is reserved for more serious complaints that cannot be resolved by local resolution.

Complaints about private dental care

The **Dental Complaints Service** comprises a team of trained advisers whose aim is to help private dental patients and dental professionals settle complaints about private dental care fairly and efficiently.

Patients may also complain directly to the General Dental Council. It is suggested that patients are more willing to complain about the care they receive from their dentist than has been the case in the past. The GDC reported that between 2010 and 2014 it experienced a 110% increase in the number of complaints from patients and members of the public, employers, other registrants and the police about GDC registrants.

Responding to a complaint

A dentist or dental care professional who receives a formal complaint should seek advice from their indemnity organization on how best to resolve the patient's complaint. Dental practices should have an in-house complaints procedure and a dedicated complaints manager.

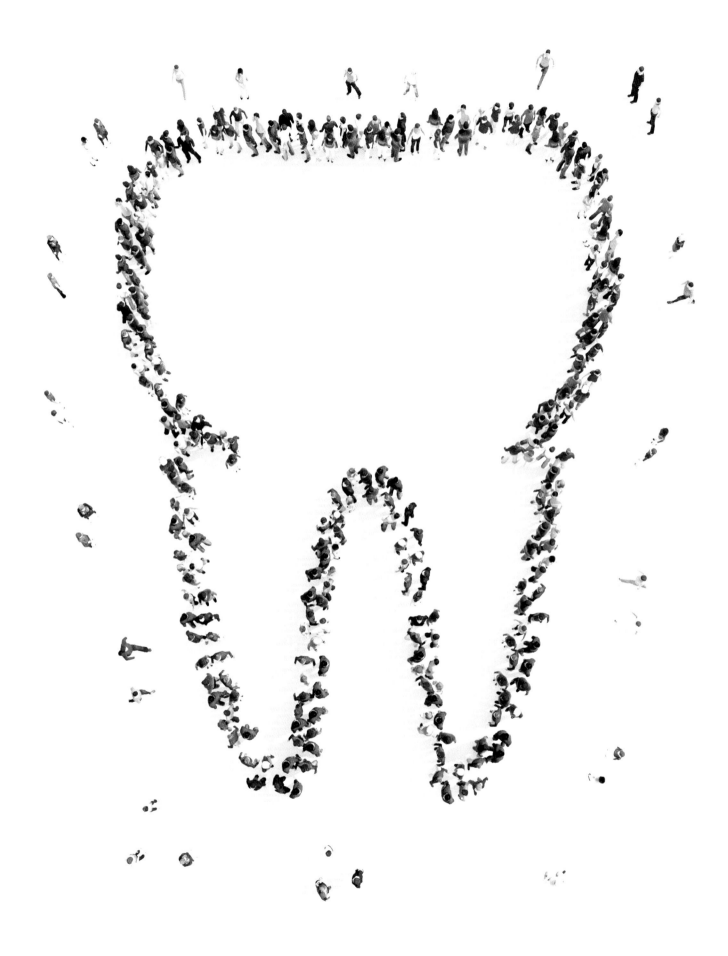

A career in dental public health

Part 12

Chapters

47 A career in dental public health

It is to be hoped that by this stage readers of this book will realize that an appreciation of oral health and dental services from a population perspective is a necessary skill for all dental professionals. The promotion of oral health at the chairside on an individual basis, and advocacy for oral health on a general level, are core components of the role of all members of the dental team.

Those working in Community Dental Services will be required to fulfil key elements of the dental public health function, such as participation in epidemiological surveys and data collection, and the organization and delivery of national or regional oral health improvement programmes.

Around the world, dental public health professionals have a key role to play in organizing the development of dental services and advocating for oral health.

Dental public health training

In the United Kingdom, dental public health is recognized as a specialty by the General Dental Council (GDC). In order to claim specialist status, a dentist must have undergone a formal programme of training, have been awarded a Certificate of Completion of Specialist Training (CCST) by the Dental Postgraduate Deanery and be on the Specialist List of the GDC.

The formal dental public health training programme in the UK lasts for four years. One year will be spent undertaking a Master's in (Dental) Public Health. A defined curriculum for dental public health specialist training has been devised by the GDC and is available on its website. Training programmes are organized by and run under the auspices of the Dental Postgraduate Deanery. The Specialist Advisory Committee in Dental Public Health of the Royal College of Surgeons of England provides quality assurance of the training programmes, although responsibility for approval lies with the Dental Postgraduate Dean.

On completion of the training programme, trainees take the Intercollegiate Specialty Fellowship Examination (ISFE) in Dental Public Health. Successful completion of this examination, together with successful completion of the training programme, enables the trainee to be awarded a CCST and thus to apply for admission to the GDC Specialist List.

Registration on the GDC Specialist List is a necessary precondition of appointment to a consultant in dental public health post in the National Health Service.

Specialists/consultants in dental public health work in two main roles. The majority are employed by Public Health England. They work with key stakeholders from a broad range of backgrounds on the improvement of oral health and delivery of dental services. The alternative role for specialists/consultants in dental public health is in academia. Here they are employed by a university and the main focus of their role is research and teaching.

Anyone interested in a career in dental public health should discuss this with their local consultant in dental public health or with the Dental Postgraduate Deanery. Alternatively, the Chairperson of the Specialist Advisory Committee in Dental Public Health can be contacted via the Royal College of Surgeons of England.

Dental Public Health at a Glance, First Edition. Ivor G. Chestnut.
© 2016 John Wiley & Sons, Ltd. Published 2016 by John Wiley & Sons, Ltd.

Ajzen, I. (1991) The theory of planned behaviour. *Organizational Behaviour and Human Decision Processes*, 50: 179–211.

Bradshaw, J.R. (1972) The taxonomy of social need. In G.McLachlan (ed.), *Problems and Progress in Medical Care*, Oxford: Oxford University Press.

Bratthall, D. (2000) Introducing the Significant Caries Index together with a proposal for a new global oral health goal for 12-year-olds. *International Dental Journal*, 50(6): 378–84.

British Fluoridation Society, http://www.bfsweb.org/ The BFS aims to encourage fluoridation of the water supply.

Cancer Research UK, www.cancerresearchuk.org/ Contains useful database on oral cancer.

Care Quality Commission (2014) *A Fresh Start for the Regulation and Inspection of Primary Care Dental Services.* http://www.cqc.org.uk/sites/default/files/fresh_start_dental_signposting_statement_august_2014.pdf

Cochrane, A. (1972) *Effectiveness and Efficiency: Random Reflections on Health Services.* Cardiff: Nuffield Provincial Hospitals Trust.

Cochrane Library, http://www.cochranelibrary.com/ The Cochrane Library is a collection of six databases that contain different types of high-quality, independent evidence to inform healthcare decision making, and a seventh database that provides information about Cochrane groups.

Cochrane Oral Health Group, http://ohg.cochrane.org/ This is an international network of healthcare professionals, researchers and consumers preparing, maintaining and disseminating systematic reviews of randomized controlled trials in oral health.

Dahlgren, G. and Whitehead, M. (1991) *Policies and Strategies to Promote Social Equity in Health.* Stockholm: Institute for Futures Studies.

Department of Health Legislation and Policy Unit, Dental and Eyecare Services (2015) *Dental Contract Reform: Prototypes, Overview Document.* https://www.gov.uk/government/uploads/system/uploads/attachment_data/file/395384/Reform_Document.pdf

Downie, R.S., Fyfe, C. and Tannahill, A. (1990) *Health Promotion: Models and Values.* Oxford: Oxford University Press.

Edwards, R. (2004) The problem of tobacco smoking. *BMJ*, 328(7433): 217–219.

General Dental Council (2013) *Scope of Practice.* http://www.gdc-uk.org/dentalprofessionals/standards/documents/scope%20of%20practice%20september%202013%20(3).pdf

General Dental Council (2014) *Facts and Figures from the GDC Register, December 2014.* http://www.gdc-uk.org/Newsandpublications/factsandfigures/Documents/Facts%20and%20figures%20from%20the%20GDC%20register%20December%202014.pdf

Greene, J.C. and Vermillion, J.R. (1960) Oral Hygiene Index: A method for classifying oral hygiene status. *Journal of the American Dental Association*, 61: 172–79.

Grossi, S.G., Zambon, J.J., Ho, A.W. et al. (1994) Assessment of risk for periodontal disease: I. Risk indicators for attachment loss. *Journal of Periodontology*, 65(3): 260–67.

Hayden, C., Bowler, J.O., Chambers, S. et al. (2014) Obesity and dental caries in children: a systematic review and meta-analysis. *Community Dentistry and Oral Epidemiology*, 41(4): 289–308. doi:10.1111/cdoe.12014

Health and Social Care Information Centre (2006) *Health Survey for England 2004: The Health of Minority Ethnic Groups.* http://www.hscic.gov.uk/catalogue/PUB01209/heal-surv-hea-eth-min-hea-tab-eng-2004-rep.pdf

Health and Social Care Information Centre, www.hscic.gov.uk/pubs/dentalsurveyfullreport09 This site gives access to the results of the 2009 Adult Dental Health Survey.

Health and Social Care Information Centre (2011) *Adult Dental Health Survey 2009 – Summary Report and Thematic Series.* http://www.hscic.gov.uk/pubs/dentalsurveyfullreport09

Health and Social Care Information Centre (2011) *Service Considerations – A Report from the Adult Dental Health Survey 2009.* http://www.hscic.gov.uk/catalogue/PUB01086/adul-dent-heal-surv-summ-them-the6-2009-rep8.pdf.

Health and Social Care Information Centre (2011) *Disease and Related Disorders: A Report from the Adult Dental Health Survey 2009.* http://www.hscic.gov.uk/catalogue/PUB01086/adul-dent-heal-surv-summ-them-the2-2009-rep4.pdf

Health and Social Care Information Centre (2014) *Improving Dental Care and Oral Health: A Call to Action.* http://www.england.nhs.uk/wp-content/uploads/2014/02/imp-dent-care.pdf.

Health and Social Care Information Centre (2014) *Improving Dental Care and Oral Health: A Call to Action Evidence Resource Pack.* http://www.england.nhs.uk/wp-content/uploads/2014/02/ dental-info-pack.pdf.

Health and Social Care Information Centre, www.hscic.gov.uk/catalogue/PUB17137 This site gives access to the results of the 2013 Dental Health Survey of Children and Young People.

Hodgson, R., Alwyn, T., John, B., Thom, B. and Smith A. (2002) The FAST alcohol screening test. *Alcohol and Alcoholism*, 37: 61–66.

Innes, N.P.T., Clarkson, J.E., Speed, C. et al. (2013) The FiCTION dental trial protocol – filling children's teeth: Indicated or not. *BMC Oral Health*, 13: 25.

Kassebaum, N.J., Bernabé, E., Dahiya, M. et al. (2014) Global burden of severe periodontitis in 1990–2010: A systematic review and meta-regression. *Journal of Dental Research*, 93(11): 1045-1053.

Kupietzky, A., Tal, E., Shapira, J. and Ram, D. (2008) Fasting state and episodes of vomiting in children receiving nitrous oxide for dental treatment. *Pediatric Dentistry*, 30(5): 414–19.

Löe, H. (1967) The gingival index, the plaque index and the retention index systems. *Journal of Periodontology*, 38(6, Suppl.): 610–16.

Marino, R.J., Khan, A.R. and Morgan, M. (2013) Systematic review of publications on economic evaluations of caries prevention programs. *Caries Research*, 47(4): 265–72.

Moher, D., Liberati, A., Tetzlaff, J., Altman, D.G. and the PRISMA Group (2009) Preferred Reporting Items for Systematic Reviews and Meta-Analyses: The PRISMA Statement. *PLoS Medicine*, 6(6): e1000097. doi:10.1371/journal.pmed1000097

National Pure Water Association, www.npwa.org.uk/ NPWA campaigns against water fluoridation.

NHS England (2014) *NHS England: A Guide to Our Vision and Purpose.* http://www.england.nhs.uk/wp-content/uploads/2014/ 06/nhse-guide-vision-purpose-2014.pdf

Nutbeam, D. (1998) Evaluating health promotion: Progress, problems and solutions. *Health Promotion International*, 13: 27–44.

Office for National Statistics (2012) *2011 Census: Population Estimates for the United Kingdom, 27 March 2011.* http://www.ons.gov.uk/ons/dcp171778_292378.pdf

Office for National Statistics (2013) *General Lifestyle Survey Overview: A Report on the 2011 General Lifestyle Survey.* http://www.ons.gov.uk/ons/rel/ghs/general-lifestyle-survey/2011/index.html

Oliveria, C.A.G.R., Dias, P.F., dos Santos, M.P.A. and Maia, L.C. (2008) Split mouth randomized controlled clinical trial of beveled cavity preparations in primary molars: An 18-Month follow up. *Journal of Dentistry*, 36: 754–8.

Prochaska, J.O. and DiClemente, C.C. (1982) Trans-theoretical therapy: Toward a more integrative model of change. *Psychotherapy: Theory, Research and Practice*, 19(3): 276–88.

Public Health England (2013) *HIV in the United Kingdom: 2013 Report* https://www.gov.uk/government/uploads/system/uploads/attachment_data/file/326601/HIV_annual_report_2013.pdf

Public Health England – Oral Health Database, www.nwph.info/dentalhealth/ Gives access to the BASCD coordinated epidemiological surveys.

Rosenstock, I.M., Strecher, V.J. and Becker, M.H. (1994) The health belief model and HIV risk behavior change. In R.J.DiClemente and J.L.Peterson (eds), *Preventing AIDS: Theories and Methods of Behavioral Intentions* (pp. 5–24). New York: Plenum Press.

Santibañez, M., Vioque, J., Alguacil, J. et al. (2008) Occupational exposures and risk of oesophageal cancer by histological type: A case-control study in eastern Spain. *Occupational and Environmental Medicine*, 65: 774–81.

Schulz, K.F., Altman, D.G. and Moher, D. for the CONSORT Group (2010) CONSORT 2010 Statement: Updated guidelines for reporting parallel group randomised trials. *BMJ*, 340: c332.

Scottish Intercollegiate Guidelines Network, www.sign.ac.uk/ Produces clinical guidelines including those of relevance to dentistry.

Scottish Intercollegiate Guidelines Network (2014) *A guideline developer's handbook.* (SIGN publication no. 50). http://www.sign.ac.uk

Scottish National Dental Inspection Programme, www.scottishdental.org/index.aspx?o=2153 Details of oral health surveys in Scotland.

Silness, J. and Löe, H. (1964) Periodontal disease in pregnancy II. *Acta Odontologica Scandinavica*, 22: 121–35.

Slade, G. (1997) Derivation and validation of a short-form oral health impact profile. *Community Dentistry and Oral Epidemiology*, 25(4): 284–90. doi:10.1111/j.1600-0528.1997.tb00941.x

Smoke-Free and Smiling, www.gov.uk/government/uploads/system/uploads/attachment_data/file/288835/SmokeFree__Smiling_110314_FINALjw.pdf This document provides updated guidance for dental teams, commissioners and educators on how they can contribute to reducing rates of tobacco use, and highlights resources available to support them.

Steele, J., Rooney, E., Clarke, J., and Wilson, T. (2009) *NHS Dental Services in England: An Independent Review Led by Professor Jimmy Steele.* London: Department of Health.

Thomson, W.M., Poulton, R., Broadbent, J.M. et al. (2008) Cannabis smoking and periodontal disease among young adults. *Journal of the American Medical Association*, 229: 525–32.

Wales Oral Health Information Unit, www.cardiff.ac.uk/dentl/research/themes/appliedclinicalresearch/epidemiology/oralhealth/index.html Details on oral health surveys in Wales.

Watt, R. (2005) Strategies and approaches in oral disease prevention and health promotion. *Bulletin of the World Health Organization*, 83: 711–18.

Welsh Government (2013) *Welsh Health Survey 2012.* http://gov.wales/docs/statistics/2013/130911-welsh-health-survey-2012-en.pdf

Wilson, J.M.G. and Jinger, G. (1968) The principles and practice of screening for disease. *Public Health Papers*, 34. Geneva: World Health Organization. http://apps.who.int/iris/bitstream/10665/37650/1/WHO_PHP_34.pdf

World Health Organization Global Oral Health Database, http://www.who.int/oral_health/databases/en/ This site gives access to the WHO's global database – it can be used to determine oral disease prevalence (where available) in countries around the world.

World Health Organization Study group on Tobacco Product Regulation (TOBREG) (2005) Advisory Note – Waterpipe tobacco smoking: Health effects, research needs and recommended action by regulators. Geneva, World Health Organisation. http://www.who.int/tobacco/global_interaction/tobreg/Waterpipe%20recommendation_Final.pdf?ua=1

World Health Organization (2015) Guideline: Sugars Intake for Adults and Children, http://www.who.int/nutrition/publications/guidelines/sugars_intake/en/ This guideline provides updated global, evidence-informed recommendations on the intake of free sugars to reduce the risk of non-communicable diseases in adults and children, with a particular focus on the prevention and control of unhealthy weight gain and dental caries.

World Health Organisation (2015), http://www.who.int/hiv/en/ [webpage]

Useful contacts and websites

British Association for the Study of Community Dentistry, www.bascd.org/ BASCD is the UK's professional association for the science, philosophy and practice of promoting the oral health of populations and groups in society.

British Dental Association, www.bda.org/ The British Dental Association (BDA) is the professional association and trade union for dentists in the United Kingdom and was founded in 1880.

Care Quality Commission, www.cqc.org.uk/ The functions of the CQC as they relate to dentistry are described in Chapter 46.

Faculty of Public Health, www.fph.org.uk/ The professional organization in the United Kingdom for generic public health.

General Dental Council, www.gdc-uk.org/Pages/default.aspx The functions of the GDC are described in Chapter 46.

National Institute for Health and Care Excellence, www.nice.org.uk/ NICE provides national guidance and advice to improve health and social care.

Public Health England, www.gov.uk/government/organisations/public-health-england An Executive Agency sponsored by the Department of Health, responsible for protecting and improving health and well-being, and reducing health inequalities.

Royal College of Surgeons of Edinburgh, www.rcsed.ac.uk/

Royal College of Surgeons of England, www.rcseng.ac.uk/ This college hosts the Specialty Advisory Committee on Dental Public Health. It also holds the Diploma in Dental Public Health Examinations.

Royal College of Physicians and Surgeons of Glasgow, www.rcpsg.ac.uk/ This College hosts the Intercollegiate Specialty Examination in Dental Public Health on behalf of all four Royal Colleges.

Royal College of Surgeons in Ireland, www.rcsi.ie/

Index

tooth staining, 73, 75
tooth wear, 18–20
toothbrushing, 15, 47
toothbrushing—school-based, 63
toothpaste, 21, 47, 58–59
toothpaste—ingredients, 59
training, 21, 35
Trans-Theoretical Model of Change, 51, 76
traumatic dental injury, 19
travellers, 87
trial—arm, 35
trial—cluster randomized controlled, 35
Tristan da Cunha, 67
Turku studies, 67
Twitter, 49

UK Border Agency, 75
units of dental activity, 97
utility measure, 93

varenicline, 77
vending machines, 49, 69
Vipeholm, 67
Vitamin C deficiency (scurvy), 67

water fluoridation, *see* fluoridation
water fluoridation—alternatives, 63
water in schools, 69
waterpipe, 75
whistleblowing, 109
WHO Global Oral Health Programme, 22
workforce, 105
World Health Organisation (WHO), 22, 29
wound healing, 73

xylitol, 69

zinc citrate, 59